CZECHOSLOVAK ACADEMY OF SCIENCES

W0049872

MYCOLOGICAL DIAGNOSIS
OF
ANIMAL DERMATOPHYTOSES

CZECHOSLOVAK ACADEMY OF SCIENCES

SCIENTIFIC EDITOR PROF. DR. KAREL CEJP
SCIENTIFIC ADVISER DOC. DR. JIŘÍ MANYCH
LANGUAGE EDITOR EVA KALINOVÁ
GRAPHIC DESIGN BY MIROSLAV HOUSKA

MYCOLOGICAL DIAGNOSIS
OF
ANIMAL DERMATOPHYTOSES

JAROSLAV DVOŘÁK • MILOŠ OTČENÁŠEK

1969

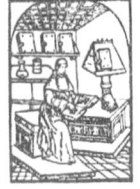

SPRINGER-SCIENCE+BUSINESS MEDIA, B.V.

ACADEMIA, PUBLISHING HOUSE
OF THE CZECHOSLOVAK ACADEMY
OF SCIENCES, PRAGUE

DISTRIBUTION THROUGHOUT THE WORLD WITH THE EXCEPTION
OF SOCIALIST COUNTRIES:

SPRINGER-SCIENCE+BUSINESS MEDIA, B.V.

ISBN 978-90-6193-236-9   ISBN 978-94-010-3426-5 (eBook)
DOI 10.1007/978-94-010-3426-5

CONTENTS

A. General

B. Special aspects

C. Techniques

LIST OF FIGURES

LIST OF PHOTOGRAPHS IN THE TEXT

1. Dermatophytic mycelium in skin scales, KOH preparation (approx. × 200).
2. Cattle hair invaded by *Trichophyton verrucosum*; KOH preparation (approx. × 500).
3. Mycelium of *T. violaceum*, iodine solution after 10 min (approx. × 250).
4. Mycelium with macroconidia of *M. gypseum*; slide culture (approx. × 100).
5. Young macroconidia of *M. gypseum*; iodine solution after 10 min (approx. × 750).
6. Mature macroconidium of *M. gypseum*; iodine solution after 10 min (approx. × 200).
7. Mycelium with macroconidia of *K. ajelloi*; slide culture (approx. × 275).
8. Mature macroconidium of *K. ajelloi*; iodine solution after 10 min (× 2,000).
9. Sessile macroconidia of *E. floccosum*; iodine solution after 10 min (× 1,500).
10. Microconidia of *T. tonsurans*; iodine solution after 10 min (approx. × 250).
11. Chlamydospores of *T. tonsurans*; iodine solution after 10 min (approx. × 250).
12. Spirals of *T. mentagrophytes*; iodine solution after 10 min (approx. × 1,000, approx. × 300).
13. Favic chandeliers of *T. verrucosum*; iodine solution after 10 min (approx. × 500).

LIST OF TABLES

PREFACE

There are not many biological disciplines, which have experienced such fast development as have human and veterinary mycology in recent years. In the initial stages organisms, whose influence on man has not been determined, have been investigated on a purely academic basis and with particular reference to their taxonomic position. As recently as the thirties, the pathogenic agents of dermatophytoses were known collectively under such names as "Microsporum" and "Trichophyton". Such designation occurred in most medical and veterinary literature irrespective of the fact that fungi are organisms of a highly complicated and most variable morphological structure, an intricate development and a distribution over a diversity of environments, infecting hosts of the animal kingdom. The greater the credit, therefore, that can be attributed to the pioneers of mycological research, the founders of modern mycology such as R. Sabouraud, M. Langeron, R. Vanbreuseghem, Ch. W. Emmons, who elucidated the importance of mycology in human and veterinary medicine. To one of them, Professor R. Vanbreuseghem, this book has been dedicated.

In spite of these tremendous efforts, many aspects of the biology and ecology of fungi have still remained obscure in view of the complicated development throughout the various phases, the variability of species and the large numbers of purely saprophytic species occurring in nature.

At the present, mycoparasitic infection in man and animals is of utmost importance. Since modern therapeutics have reduced the incidence of various bacterioses and rickettsioses and some viral diseases have been controlled by successful vaccination, increased interest has been taken in fungal diseases. Even the highest medical and veterinary organisations of the UNO focussed their attention on these problems. At the meeting of the WHO and FAO Committee of Experts on Zoonoses, held at the end of 1966 in Geneva, the importance of these problems was stressed by the demand for further research in the field of dermatophytoses and systemic mycoses. This shows the great need of intensified research in medical and veterinary mycology, conducted at various levels.

For these reasons the book "Mycological diagnosis of animal dermato-phytoses", presented by J. Dvořák and M. Otčenášek of the Institute of Parasitology, Czechoslovak Academy of Sciences, Prague and concerned with the various aspects of animal dermatophytoses, should be most welcomed.

The authors have laid down solid foundations for the mycological diag-nosis of dermatophytoses in veterinary practice, a problem until now very little discussed in world literature. They present fundamental knowledge on the morphology, development and ecology of fungi, collected over a period of more than 15 years of active work and study. Their experiences in human my-cology have been applied successfully in veterinary mycology.

The book is divided into three parts. Part One is an introduction to the study of dermatophytes as animal parasites, giving information on standard methods of cultivation and identification. Part Two reviews the species in-fecting animals; Part Three discusses techniques, which should be used for the exact identification of dermatophytes.

The authors have tried to give an accurate picture of fungi that cause infection in animals, by reference to all aspects of contemporary taxonomy, biology and ecology.

By recording the results obtained in mycoparasitology of dermatophytes in Czechoslovakia and the other socialist countries and confronting them with the most important achievements in the capitalist countries, the book may be of valuable help by presenting a complete picture on the present state of mycoparasitological research in the world.

After World War II mycology, following a general world trend, started to be developed in Czechoslovakia. This was done on several levels. In view of the general lay-out of this book, I shall outline this development principally with regard to medical and veterinary mycology.

The first systematic study concerned with human dermatophytology, based on 115 isolations of dermatophytes from man during the years 1933 to 1936 and on their detailed study, was published by OBRTEL (Prague 1936) under the title: "Les caractéristiques morphologiques et biologiques des teignes de la peau se présentant à Prague". Even today, this book has retained its basic value. The Atlas of Dermatophytes, published by the same author in 1950, offers an excellent aid for the diagnosis of these fungi. In 1946, CHMEL recorded a list of dermatophytes isolated from human lesions in 1942—1946. His recent book on dermatophytoses of man and their treatment (CHMEL 1964) also deserves to be mentioned. FRÁGNER (1958) published a most useful monograph on this subject, reviewing his longlasting experiences in the labora-tory. A more recent publication by HÜBSCHMANN and FRÁGNER (1962) on der-matophytes and skin diseases caused by them, also merits attention.

Shortly after World War II, mycoparasitological laboratories were set up in Prague (Manych — Laboratory for Medical Mycology) and Olomouc (Hejtmánek, Hejtmánková – Biological Institute of the Faculty of Medicine).

In 1947, research on dermatophytes was started at the Dermatophytological Laboratory of the Faculty of Medicine at Hradec Králové under the leadership of Prof. Fingerland and Prof. Janoušek, later under Prof. Málek.

As it would be most difficult to name all prominent Czech and Slovak mycologists I shall record only those, whose work has inspired the senior author of this book, Dr. Dvořák, to study medical mycology, particularly myco-parasitology of homoiothermous animals. In the first place the excellent publication by CORDA (1837–1854), custodian of the National Museum in Prague, entitled: "Icones fungorum hucusque cognitorum" and, in recent years "Houby" (Fungi) by CEJP (1957), an important textbook on parasitic fungi and fungi in general, now recognized as one of the fundaments of mycological research in Czechoslovakia.

Dr. Dvořák started mycological work at the Dermatophytological Laboratory of the Faculty of Medicine at Hradec Králové in 1949. In 1954, he published with Dočekal the "Manual of Medical Mycology" (DOČEKAL and DVOŘÁK 1954). Some years later, this laboratory concerned with the diagnosis of dermatophytoses in eastern Bohemia, was moved to Pardubice. In 1962 the mycological group of the Institute of Parasitology of the Czechoslovak Academy of Sciences was established and there, the author continued in his work in close collaboration with the second author of this book, Dr. Otčenášek. The interest of both authors in animal dermatophytes was fostered by Prof. Sova and Dr. Komárek of the Veterinary Hospital at Pardubice who gave them the opportunity to examine animals, especially cattle and horses, on a more extensive scale. Later they were asked to take over mycological control of large breeding stocks of laboratory animals at Rosice n/Labem (Research Institute for Pharmacy and Biochemistry, Director Dr. Hradil).

Dr. Dvořák and Dr. Otčenášek, having devoted years to the study of dermatophytes, are now presenting the results of their patient and long-lasting work for the benefit of all those, who may use their book in practice to add to their efficiency and economy of time.

It is hardly necessary to emphasize that every biologist, regardless of his specialisation, should know the organism with which he is working. Such knowledge is expected ever more from veterinarians and physicians, especially, if the pathogenic agent causes infection in man and animals. The excellent arrangement of the book allows every user to identify the taxonomic position, even as far as the species, of every dermatophyte isolated from any domestic animal.

Prof. Dr. B. Rosický, DSc.

Corresponding Member of the Czechoslovak
Academy of Sciences
Director of the Institute of Parasitology, Prague

Acknowledgments

We are very indebted to Dr. J. Komárek of the Veterinary Hospital at Pardubice for the list of clinical characteristics of dermatophytoses. All photographs were contributed by Dr. Z. Hubálek, a member of our team, to whom we are happy to acknowledge our indebtedness. We also wish to thank Dr. J. Kunert from the Biological Institute of the Faculty of Medicine, Palacký University, Olomouc for his valuable advice and help in the elaboration of the part concerned with perfect states of dermatophytes. For valuable technical assistance special thanks are given to ·Mrs. E. Blehová, H. Dyntarová, E. Kalinová, M. Králová and J. Kuchařová from the Institute of Parasitology, Czechoslovak Academy of Sciences, Prague, to V. Jaroměřský and A. Ličbinská from the District Station of Hygiene and Epidemiology, Pardubice and to Dr. J. Holda, Institute for Pharmacy and Biochemistry, Rosice n/Labem.

For the provision or identification of dermatophytes and Chrysosporia and other valuable information, we express our thanks to: V. A. Balabanoff (Sofia), J. Buchvald (Bratislava), J. M. Doby (Rennes), Mrs. M. Doby-Dubois (Rennes), R. Evolceanu (Bucharest), E. Flórián (Budapest), D. Frey (Sydney), L. K. Georg (Atlanta), D. Hantschke (Essen), M. Hejtmánek (Olomouc), N. Hejtmánková (Olomouc), Z. Herpay (Debrecen), J. Manych (Prague), L. Ožegović (Sarajevo), H. Paldrok (Stockholm), J. A. Rioux (Montpellier), Ch. Schönborn (Leipzig), R. Vanbreuseghem (Antwerp).

A. GENERAL

INTRODUCTION

For the study of the epizootology and epidemiology of animal dermatophytoses, identification of the dermatophyte is of fundamental importance. This is especially important if specific antimycotic agents are available.

The relative importance of animal dermatophytoses has appeared to increase during the last decade. The incidence of other more seriously damaging animal diseases has been reduced and more attention has been paid to diseases of mycotic origin. It must be noted that many animal dermatophytoses may be transmitted to man.

The mycological diagnosis of dermatophytoses is dependent on knowledge of the taxonomy of dermatophytes. The identification procedure attempts to reveal specific differentiating characters. Incidentally, the diagnostic procedure suggests corrections in taxonomy. New methods allow the recognition of new characters and it is necessary to ascertain the diagnostic significance of these characters, their stability and also, whether they are in accord with the present concepts of dermatophytes.

Todays concepts of dermatophytes cannot be considered to be definite. In general, all mycologists have a particular interest in determining species by biological (genotypical, phylogenetical) means.

In our opinion, the system of classification submitted by Georg on the occasion of the IXth International Congress of Dermatology in Stockholm, 1957 and all the systems subsequently accepted, do not, in fact, allow the determination of species.

Thirty years ago it seemed that reliable methods to differentiate species were available. DAVIDSON, DOWDING and BULLER (1932) concluded that hyphal fusion (anastomoses) developed easily between mycelia cf the same species but, on the contrary, that heterospecific hyphae did not produce anastomoses. Therefore, each atypical strain isolated can be identified if its anastomosing capacity with all typical dermatophyte species is examined. Then, this isolate is conspecific (of identical species) with the anastomosing dermatophyte. DVOŘÁK (1957) demonstrated that anastomoses develop even between different species. HEJTMÁNEK (1959) confirmed this observed phenomenon. BENEDEK (1964) reported hyphal fusion between *Keratinomyces ajelloi* and *Microsporon gypseum* and concluded that these dermatophytes, though morphologically different, are biochemically conspecific. At the present time, this method is considered unreliable when used in diagnosis or in the establishment of true species.

It is possible that a more intensive and extensive study of antigenic structure can be helpful in establishing valid species. In 1937, it was shown that the following dermatophytes differ in their antigenic structure (after WILDFÜHR 1961):

	Presence of antigenic components		
Trichophyton mentagrophytes	A	B	G
T. m. var. *interdigitale*	A	—	KW
T. m. var. *quinckeanum*	A	B	Q
T. schoenleinii	—	—	SCH

Recently, perfect states of many dermatophytes, especially those which live primarily in soil, have been discovered. Also these studies can help in the elucidation of these problems.

At present HEJTMÁNEK et al. (1967) are studying the properties of induced mutants. Such investigations, electronoptic, cytogenetic and other studies can be of great value for these problems.

Without any doubt, at the present time, such an artificial classification can be established only after the phenotypical characters of dermatophytes have been examined in culture under defined standard conditions.

To submit exhaustive and precise rules for diagnosis based on present day concepts of dermatophytes is not easy. The dermatophytes are variable organisms, the appearance of their morpho-physiological properties is largely dependent upon cultivation conditions, upon the host etc. Today, nobody is able to take all considerations into account and, therefore, some strains must remain unidentified — e.g. *Trichophyton* sp.

A second very important problem is the estimation of the significance of dermatophytes found in the lesions.

Especially recently many dermatophytes have been isolated from the apparently healthy skin of various animals (OTČENÁŠEK and DVOŘÁK 1962 a.o.). Therefore, the possibility must be considered that a dermatophytosis-like lesion can be contaminated by dermatophytes.

Especially from human lesions often two and sometimes three different dermatophytes have been isolated simultaneously. Recently, various combinations have been recorded by DVOŘÁK and OTČENÁŠEK (1966).

The term mixed or simultaneous infection is used for the designation of such a case where from one, well circumscribed lesion, two or even more different dermatophytes are isolated.

Especially in human dermatophytology simultaneous examination of two different lesions (e.g. tinea corporis and tinea pedis) sometimes indicates two different dermatophytes (e.g. *T. verrucosum* and *T. rubrum*). Such cases are designated concurrent infections.

If one single lesion is repeatedly examined by cultivation, in rare cases first one dermatophyte is found and later another. In these cases the term consecutive infection is used.

In these cases, however, the use of the term infection is not entirely correct. It is possible that both infective agents colonize the locality simultaneously and that the result is obtained because inefficient isolation methods have been used.

Even if two dermatophytes have a real etiological role, the possibility exists that sometimes only one of them is isolated and designated as the cause.

Today, no reliable method exists for the estimation of the causal role of the dermatophyte isolated. The following criteria may, however, assist:

1. a single dermatophyte grows from several inoculated particles,
2. the same dermatophyte (and not another) is isolated from several inocula after repeated examination of the lesion,
3. the material contains typical parasitic microscopical elements of dermatophytes (hyaline, septate, branching hyphae and spores).

I. HISTORICAL NOTES

Remak probably observed for the first time that in the so-called favic scutula, filamentous elements apparently of fungous nature are present. Many years ago, Schönlein directed attention to the causal role of these mould filaments. He wrote "... und gleich die ersten Versuche liessen keinen Zweifel über die Pilznatur der sogenannten Pusteln". Gruby may have been the first to have verified the fungous etiology of some skin lesions. Sabouraud, one of the most important pioneers of dermatophytology, has paid tribute as follows: "Gruby est l'homme, qui découvrit l'origine mycosique de toutes les teignes humaines" (SABOURAUD 1910). The first dermatophytological discoveries arose from studies of human diseases. Progress in knowledge of animal dermatophytoses began later and was slow up to the present time in spite of the relatively great importance of them not only for veterinary, but also for human medicine, because animal dermatophytoses are often transmitted to man.

II. THE TERM DERMATOPHYTOSIS

This term may be reserved for the designation of such diseases as are caused by the parasitic and pathogenic activity of dermatophytes, by metabolism, growth and reproduction of these fungi directly in host tissue. Dermatophytoses are therefore true mycoses of keratinized structures of homoiothermous animals including man. Dermatophytoses are known under various names in human and veterinary medicine. Information concerning dermatophytoses occurs frequently in articles where the term dermatomycosis is used in the same sense. However, dermatomycoses may include not only dermatophytoses but also other mycoses of the skin and its appendages. Entirely corresponding is the term dermatophytia. The names ringworm or tinea have approximately the same meaning. Frequently, a more precise designation of the dermatophytosis is obtained after consideration of the clinical picture or its etiology. Here belong the terms favus, microsporia and trichophytia. In both animal and human medicine also other names circulate (e.g. herpes tonsurans). The designation dermatophytosis is useful especially for a mycologist. It has a single disadvantage — this name signifies for some human dermatologists a special type of this mycosis. Now it is necessary to clarify the meaning of the term dermatophytes. Dermatophytes are mould-like fungi arranged among *Deuteromycetes* (classis), *Moniliales* (ordo). Here they form a family, *Dermatophytaceae* (NOVÁK and GALGÓCZY 1963).

III. THE TAXONOMY OF DERMATOPHYTES

The taxonomy of dermatophytes still attracts the attention of medical mycologists. Almost 10 years ago, at the International Congress of Dermatology in Stockholm (1957), GEORG submitted a system of classification which consisted of 16 species:

A. *Microsporum* Gruby (1843)
   1. *M. audouinii* Gruby (1843)
   2. *M. canis* Bodin (1902)
   3. *M. gypseum* (Bodin) Guiart et Grigorakis (1928)

B. *Trichophyton* Malmsten (1845)
   1. *T. concentricum* Blanchard (1896)
   2. *T. equinum* (Matruchot et Dassonville) Gedoelst (1902)
   3. *T. ferrugineum* (Ota) Langeron et Milochevitch (1930)
   4. *T. gallinae* (Mégnin) Silva et Benham (1952)
   5. *T. megninii* Blanchard (1896)
   6. *T. mentagrophytes* (Robin) Blanchard (1896)
   7. *T. rubrum* (Castellani) Sabouraud (1911)
   8. *T. schoenleinii* (Lebert) Langeron et Milochevitch (1930)
   9. *T. sudanense* Joyeux (1912)
   10. *T. tonsurans* Malmsten (1845)
   11. *T. verrucosum* Bodin (1902)
   12. *T. violaceum* Sabouraud apud Bodin (1902)

C. *Epidermophyton* Sabouraud (1910)
   1. *E. floccosum* (Harz) Langeron et Milochevitch (1930)

Many dermatophytes described up till 1957 have been arranged as synonyms. In our opinion the position of *M. equinum* Bodin, 1896, *T. sulphureum* Fox, 1908, *T. persicolor* Sabouraud, 1910, *Sabouraudites duboisi* Vanbreuseghem, 1949, *T. rodhainii* Vanbreuseghem, 1949, *S. langeronii* Vanbreuseghem, 1950, *S. praecox* Rivalier, 1954 is not very clear. In the 10 years after the Congress several new dermatophyte species have been described: *M. cookei* Ajello, 1959, *T. kuryangei* Vanbreuseghem et Rosenthal, 1961, *Thallomicrosporon kuehnii* Benedek, 1963, *M. vanbreuseghemii* Georg, Ajello, Friedman et Brinkman, 1962, *M. rivalierii* Vanbreuseghem, 1963, *Keratino-myces longifusus* Flórián et Galgóczy, 1964, *T. georgii* Varsavsky et Ajello, 1964, *T. vanbreuseghemii* Rioux, Jarry et Juminer, 1964, *M. racemosum* Borelli, 1965. Of these species *M. cookei* and *M. vanbreuseghemii* have been repeatedly reported by various authors and their perfect states recognized. Therefore, they merit attention. It seems that *T. kuryangei* is an African form of *T. megninii*. *T. evolceanui* and *T. indicum* probably do not belong among dermatophytes. The remaining dermatophytes described have not till now been repeatedly isolated by other authors. From previously described dermato-phytes which have not been included in the system of Georg, the following dermatophytes are repeatedly reported and their validity as species agreed: *M. fulvum* Uriburu, 1909, *T. gourvilii* Catanei, 1933, *Keratinomyces ajelloi* Vanbreuseghem, 1952, *M. distortum* di Menna et Marples, 1954, *M. nanum* Fuentes, 1956, *T. terrestre* Durie et Frey, 1957, *T. yaoundei* Cochet, Doby-Dubois, Deblock, Doby et Vaiva, 1957 and *T. simii* (Pinoy), Stockdale, Macken-zie et Austwick, 1965. It must be noted also that the perfect states of *K. ajelloi*, *M. nanum*, *T. simii* and *T. terrestre* have been recognized.

Recently, *T. ferrugineum* has been transferred to the genus *Microsporon* (it has been recommended to use the name *Microsporon* and not *Microsporum* — see Benedek T.: Mycopath. Mycol. Appl. 19, 269—270, 1963). We consider the following dermatophytes to be valid species.

A. *Epidermophyton* Sabouraud, 1910

    1. *E. floccosum* (Harz) Langeron et Milochevitch, 1930

B. *Keratinomyces* Vanbreuseghem, 1952

    2. *K. ajelloi* Vanbreuseghem, 1952

C. *Microsporon* Gruby, 1843

    3. *M. audouinii* Gruby, 1843
    4. *M. canis* Bodin, 1902
    5. *M. cookei* Ajello, 1959
    6. *M. distortum* di Menna et Marples, 1954
    7. *M. ferrugineum* Ota, 1922
    8. *M. fulvum,* Uriburu, 1909
    9. *M. gypseum* (Bodin) Guiart et Grigorakis, 1928
    10. *M. nanum* Fuentes, 1956
    11. *M. vanbreuseghemii* Georg, Ajello, Friedman et Brinkman, 1962

D. *Trichophyton* Malmsten, 1845

   12. *T. concentricum* Blanchard, 1896
   13. *T. equinum* (Matruchot et Dassonville) Gedoelst, 1902
   14. *T. gallinae* (Mégnin) Silva et Benham, 1952
   15. *T. gourvilii* Catanei, 1933
   16. *T. megninii* Blanchard, 1896
   17. *T. mentagrophytes* (Robin) Blanchard, 1896
   18. *T. rubrum* (Castellani) Sabouraud, 1911
   19. *T. schoenleinii* (Lebert) Langeron et Milochevitch, 1930
   20. *T. simii* (Pinoy), Stockdale, Mackenzie et Austwick, 1965
   21. *T. sudanense* Joyeux, 1912
   22. *T. terrestre* Durie et Frey, 1957
   23. *T. tonsurans* Malmsten, 1845
   24. *T. verrucosum* Bodin, 1902
   25. *T. violaceum* Sabouraud apud Bodin, 1902
   26. *T. yaoundei* Cochet, Doby-Dubois, Deblock et Vaiva, 1957

A comparison of two older classification systems of dermatophytes with the recent one by Georg is shown on Tab. 1. In the ten-year period (1957—1967), 13 perfect states of 10 dermatophytes have been described (see Tab. 20).

International Code of Nomenclature

It must be stated that some authors are not respecting the International Bacteriological Code of Nomenclature (J. Gen. Microbiol. 3 : 444—462, 1949) and the International Code of the Botanical Congress (Paris, 1954, 5th Ed., Utrecht, 1955) so that some extremely important studies lose their value.

HEJTMÁNEK (1966) published the most important principles essential for every one studying dermatophytologic taxonomy. We consider it useful to give a brief and modified extract of these principles.

1. The International Code of Nomenclature regulates the use of names of taxons (taxonomic units as varieties and genera).
2. The constitution of taxons is the object of scientific research; the nomenclature takes care only of the names.
3. Each taxon must have only one correct name.
4. One single name must be used for each taxon.
5. It is not permitted to change any correct name.
6. It is necessary to change the name if it is definitely incorrect.
7. If several names exist for a single taxon, only one name corresponding with the Code must be selected and the others recorded as synonyms.
8. If a single name exists for several taxons, this name must be reserved for the first taxon designated as such.

9. Well established incorrect names must not be changed if they are sanctioned by the International Congress.
10. The name of a taxon is a pure symbol and must not express any distinct or special property.
11. A new name must be accompanied by a Latin diagnosis and by a note expressing the kind of the taxon (variety, species, genus).
12. The name of each taxon is permanently joined to the nomenclatoric type, to the concrete culture or, in higher taxons (e.g. genus), to a subordinated unit, which is in a certain sense typical for the corresponding higher taxon.
13. It must be expected that the results of taxonomic studies may change the taxonomic values, arrangement and nomenclature.

IV. THE IMPORTANCE OF INDIVIDUAL DERMATOPHYTES FOR VETERINARY MEDICINE

Individual dermatophytes are of different importance in the light of contemporary knowledge of veterinary medicine. The following are clearly pathogenic only for man: *M. ferrugineum, T. concentricum. T. gourvilii, T. sudanense* and *T. yaoundei. E. floccosum,* previously considered to be an anthropophilic, obligatory parasite of man, has been isolated recently from the mouse. *T. terrestre* seems to be geophilic, not pathogenic for homoiothermous animals. *K. ajelloi* and *M. cookei,* which also are geophilic, only exceptionally attack animals. *M. audouinii, T. megninii, T. rubrum, T. schoenleinii, T. tonsurans* and *T. violaceum* are known mainly to be human parasites, animal infections being reported only occasionally. *M. distortum* and *M. vanbreuseghemii* cannot be classified up till the present from this point of view. The remaining species, on the contrary, are very important for the veterinarian, because they often attack animals. The host range of the individual dermatophytes is given in Tab. 2.

V. THE LOCATION OF HUMAN DERMATOPHYTIC LESIONS

As mentioned above, sometimes animal dermatophytoses are transmitted to man and vice versa. Therefore, the location of human lesions caused by the individual dermatophyte species, is given in Tab. 3. The frequent infection of the same part of the human body is explained, in part, by the susceptibility to exposure, but to a greater extent, by the adaptation of the dermatophyte to certain environmental conditions, e.g. humidity and temperature. Some dermatophytes are well known and frequently isolated so that their affinity for various parts of the human body can be relatively precisely estimated. *E. floccosum*, e.g., most frequently causes tinea cruris, while *M. audouinii* is well adapted for parasitic life in the scalps of children. *T. rubrum* is very often isolated from the interdigital folds of feet, but commonly also from the perigenital region. With the exception of tinea capitis and barbae, which it causes only rarely, it can frequently be isolated from various parts of the body including the nails. It seems to be the most frequent cause of tinea unguium.

VI. THE PROPAGATION OF DERMATOPHYTES UNDER NATURAL CONDITIONS

Some dermatophytes are known as free-living saprophytes in nature. E.g. *T. terrestre* has up to the present time been known only as a saprophyte living probably in the soil. *K. ajelloi*, *M. cookei*, *M. gypseum* and *M. nanum* also

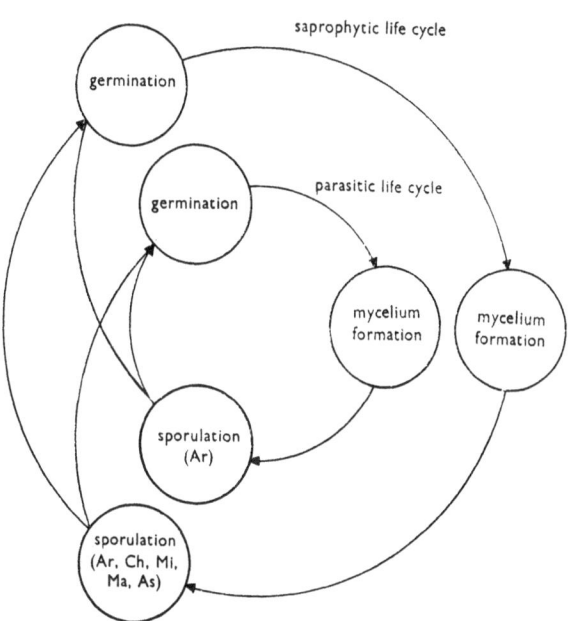

Fig. 1. Life cycles of dermatophytes under natural conditions (Ar — arthrospores, As — ascospores, Ch — chlamydospores, Ma — macroconidia, Mi — microconidia).

probably live primarily as soil saprophytes, but are capable of parasitic life. All other dermatophytes up till the present have been known only as parasites of animals and man and their saprophytic mode of life is known only under laboratory conditions. Fig. 1 shows schematically the life cycles of all dermato-

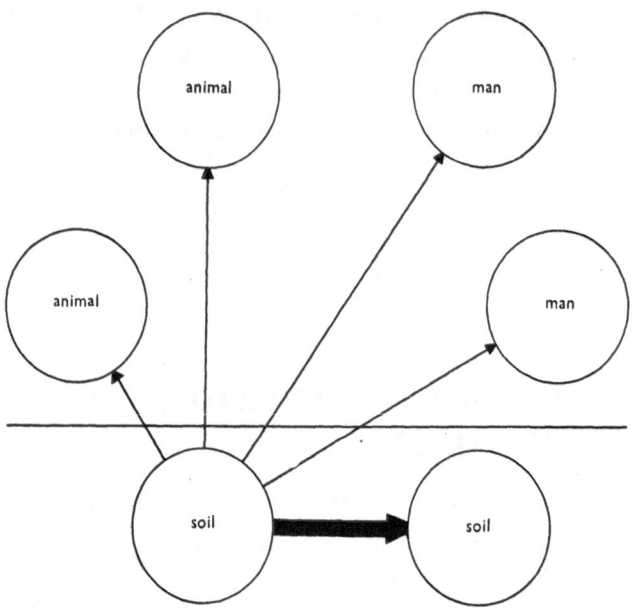

Fig. 2. Propagation modes of geophilic dermatophytes
(*K. ajelloi, M. cookei, M. gypseum/M. fulvum, M. nanum*).

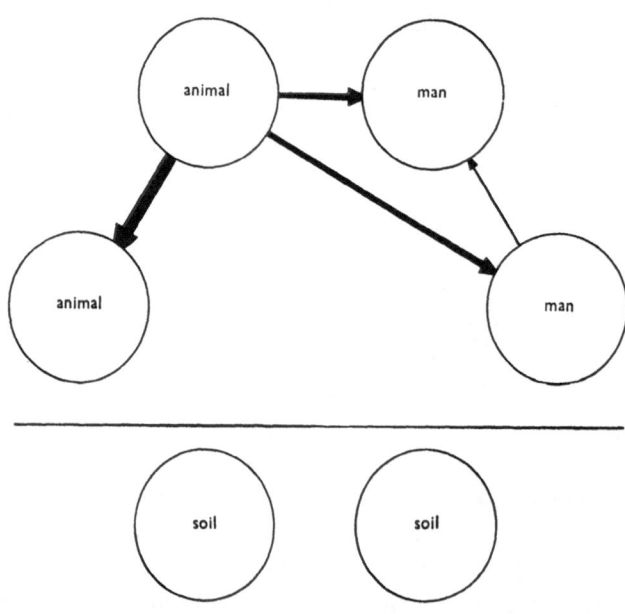

Fig. 3. Propagation modes of zoophilic dermatophytes commonly infecting man (*M. canis, T. verrucosum*).

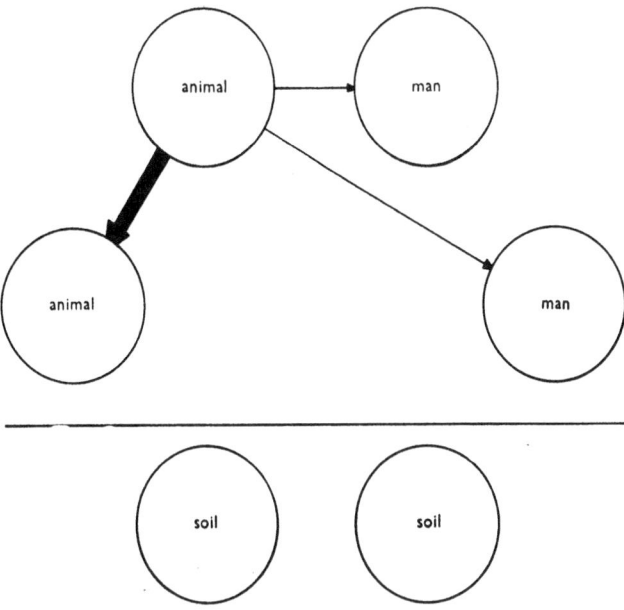

Fig. 4. Propagation modes of zoophilic dermatophytes occasionally infecting man (*T. equinum*, *T. gallinae*).

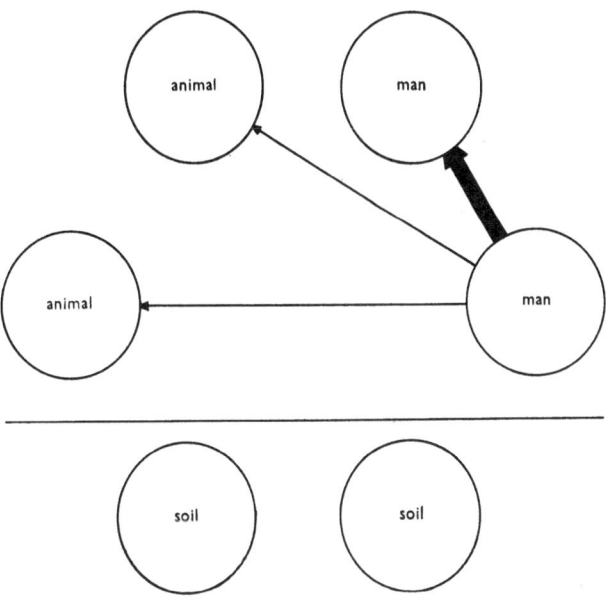

Fig. 5. Propagation modes of anthropophilic dermatophytes occasionally infecting animals (*E. floccosum*, *M. audouinii*, *T. rubrum*, *T. schoenleinii*, *T. violaceum*).

phytes according to present day knowledge. It must be mentioned that perfect states are known in all so-called geophilic or terrestrial dermatophytes. In the course of their soil saprophytism they are generally capable of producing arthrospores, chlamydospores, microconidia, macroconidia and ascospores, while in the course of parasitic life all dermatophytes produce only arthrospores. It must be added that probably all spores produced by pathogenic geophilic dermatophytes during their soil saprophytism are able to germinate, to form a mycelium, which arthrosporulates when a susceptible organism has been infected. Arthrospores produced in the course of parasitic life can infect other susceptible organisms. Evidently, this process of host-to-host transmission can be repeated. However, sometimes these arthrospores contaminate the soil and a saprophytic perfect and/or imperfect state of life and sporulation can start. Parasitic dermatophytes, which are not known as free-living saprophytes, repeat only the cycle arthrospore-arthrospore. This conception is preliminary but corresponding with present day knowledge. From these viewpoints, the dermatophytes may be divided into three groups:

1. Saprophytic cycle of propagation only — *T. terrestre*.
2. Propagation mainly during the course of saprophytism, infection of animals and man only occasional. Repetition of parasitic cycle or return of parasitic elements to the soil unusual — *K. ajelloi, M. cookei, M. fulvum/M. gypseum, M. nanum*.
3. All other dermatophytes repeat their parasitic cycle. No substrate of their intercurrent saprophytism is known up till the present.

It may be useful to demonstrate the main ways of propagation of dermatophytes, which infect animals.

1. *K. ajelloi, M. cookei, M. fulvum/M. gypseum* and *M. nanum* are frequently found in the soil. They infect only occasionally animals and man. The main source of these infections is the soil (Fig. 2) and probably hairs of the so-called carriers (these dermatophytes are commonly isolated from the hair of apparently healthy animals).
2. *M. canis* and *T. verrucosum* probably primarily live on animals, interanimal transmission is the most common method of propagation. Infection of man is common and mainly of animal origin (Fig. 3).
3. *T. equinum* and *T. gallinae* probably also primarily propagate among animals. Occasional infections of man are of animal origin (Fig. 4).
4. *E. floccosum, M. audouinii, T. rubrum, T. schoenleinii* and *T. violaceum* probably primarily propagate in the human population. Occasional infection of animals is of human origin (Fig. 5).

VII. GEOGRAPHICAL DISTRIBUTION OF DERMATOPHYTES

In Table 4 a survey of the known continental distribution of individual dermatophytes is given. Some dermatophytes (e. g. *M. vanbreuseghemii*) have been only rarely reported. Their apparent absence from other countries may be due to incorrect identification. The examination of soil for the presence of dermatophytes has been intensively carried out especially in the U.S.A. and in Europe. Immense areas of Africa and Asia remain entirely unexplored. This survey, in fact, is far from complete.

VIII. THE PRESENT DAY CONCEPT OF DERMATOPHYTES

Dermatophytes have been divided by AJELLO (1962) into two groups. The first group includes anthropophilic, zoophilic and geophilic cosmopolitan species and the second group anthropophilic and zoophilic species with a limited geographical distribution. DVOŘÁK and OTČENÁŠEK (1964) attempted to consolidate his original suggestions in the light of recent work. Table 5 shows the present day concept of the authors.

IX. DIAGNOSTIC CHARACTERS OF DERMATOPHYTES

Two fundamental methods for mycological diagnosis of a dermatophytosis are used — direct microscopy and cultivation.

Keratinous material removed from a suspected lesion (skin scales, crusts, hairs, quills, feathers) must always be examined by both methods to determine the presence of dermatophytes.

X. DIRECT MICROSCOPY

The microscopical examination of specimens enables prompt confirmation of the clinical diagnosis of dermatophytosis. Its advantage is that it is simple, easy to perform and, particularly, it can be accomplished within a short time. Its disadvantage is limited reliability: specimens taken from animal lesions sometimes contain a great amount of dried exudate which hampers the examination of preparations.

The parasitic elements must be searched for by the use of direct microscopy. Parasitic elements of dermatophytes are hyphae and arthrospores. The hyphae are usually branching, septate, hyaline tubes measuring 2—4 μm in diameter and containing protoplasm. The spores produced in the lesions and also on the surface of hairs, are probably all of the arthrospore type, developing by fragmentation of the hyphae. They can, therefore, remain arranged in chains. They are cylindrical to spherical measuring 2—10 μm. In skin scrapings (scales) it has not been possible to identify reliably the species of dermato-

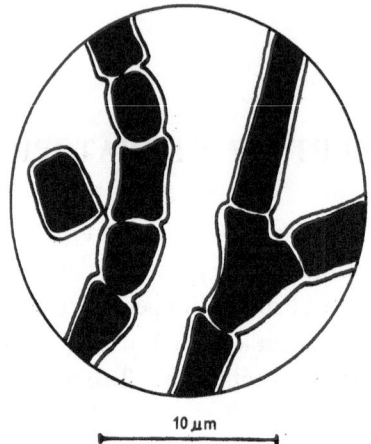

Fig. 6. Dermatophytic elements in skin scrapings.

10 μm

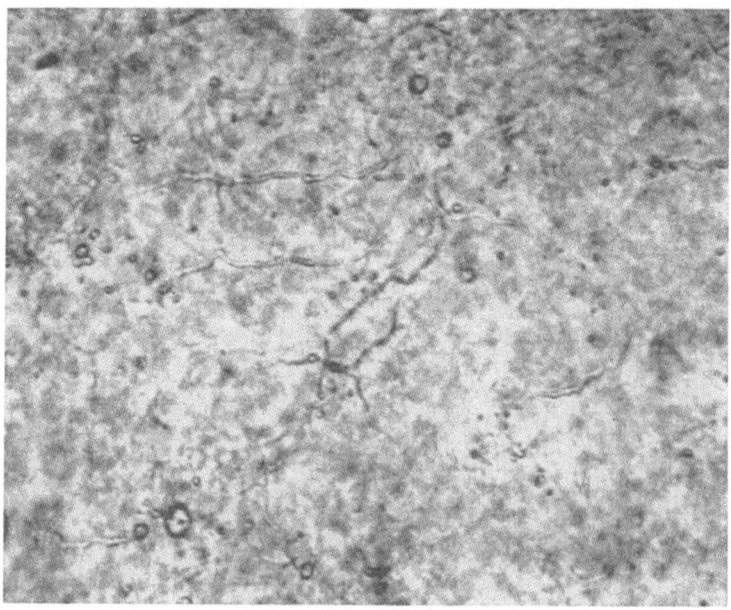

Phot. 1. Dermatophytic mycelium in skin scales, KOH preparation, (approx. × 200).

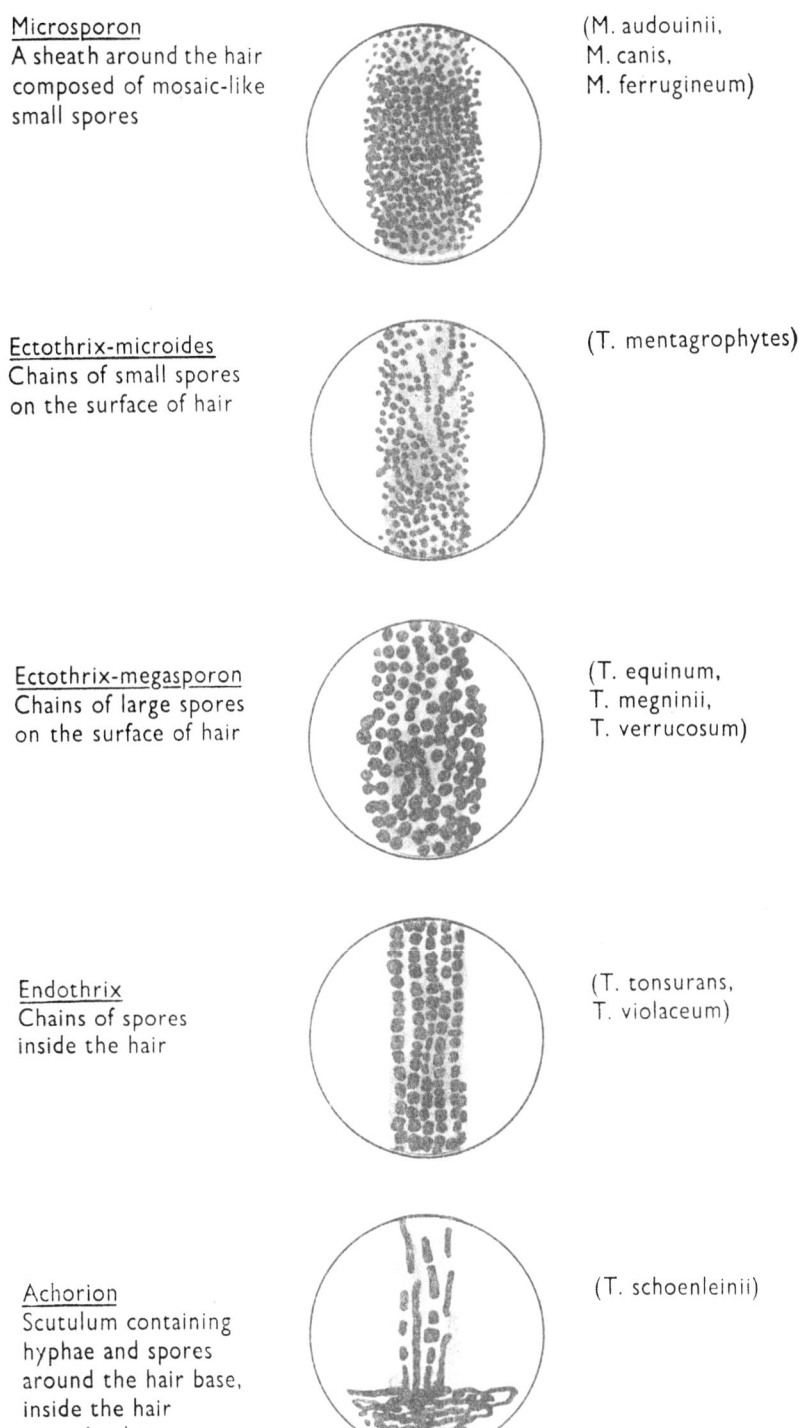

Microsporon
A sheath around the hair
composed of mosaic-like
small spores

(M. audouinii,
M. canis,
M. ferrugineum)

Ectothrix-microides
Chains of small spores
on the surface of hair

(T. mentagrophytes)

Ectothrix-megasporon
Chains of large spores
on the surface of hair

(T. equinum,
T. megninii,
T. verrucosum)

Endothrix
Chains of spores
inside the hair

(T. tonsurans,
T. violaceum)

Achorion
Scutulum containing
hyphae and spores
around the hair base,
inside the hair
some hyphae

(T. schoenleinii)

Fig. 7. Modes of hair invasion in vivo (formerly used division of dermatophytes).

phytes. However, almost always, the finding of more or less arthrosporulated hyphae permits the diagnosis of a dermatophytosis (see Fig. 6 and Photo 1).

The second most frequently examined specimens are hairs. As compared with the examination of lesions, the examination of hair sometimes permits an approximate group diagnosis. For the selection of infected hairs, the use of Wood's lamp (see C II) can sometimes be useful. The hairs parasitized by some dermatophytes fluoresce and, when such fluorescent hairs are examined (by microscopy and cultivation), the results are excellent. The survey reported in Table 6 shows that this method itself can be of valuable aid in diagnosis.

The significance of microscopical examination of hairs invaded in vivo by dermatophytes has been overestimated. It is necessary to point out that the manifestation of the interaction between two living organisms can widely vary.

The dermatophytes have been divided into several groups according to the way they parasitize hair (see Fig. 7).

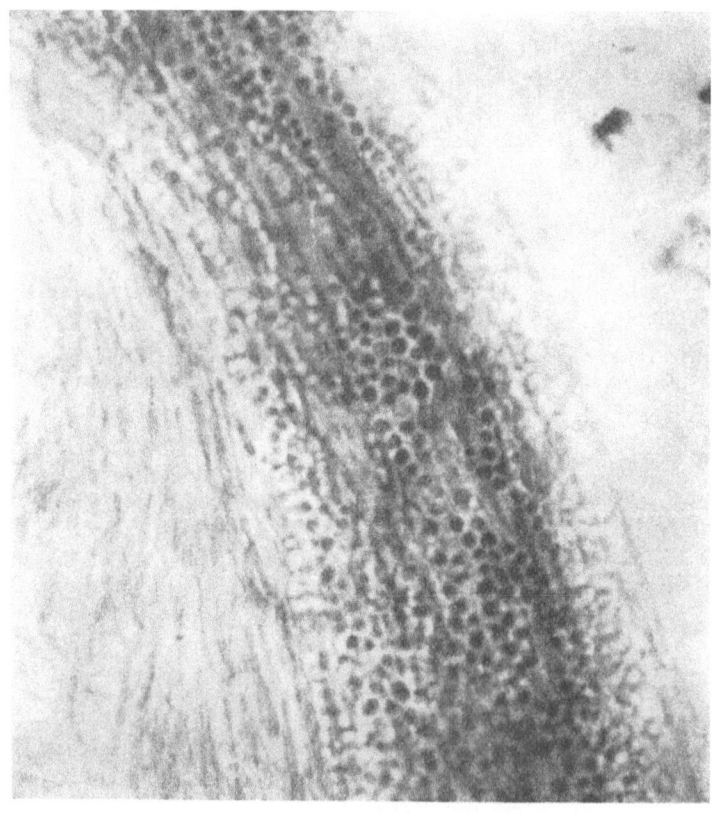

Phot. 2. Cattle hair invaded by *Trichophyton verrucosum*; KOH preparation (approx. × 500).

34

Favic scutulum is a yellow crust lenticular in shape with a depression above. Its hyphae and spores form a ring round the follicular orifice. This ring often attains the size of a pea or is even bigger (after DODGE 1935). Similar scutula can be formed round the feather (*T. gallinae*). The microsporon and ectothrix type of hair invasion is called by some authors the endoectothrix type (with small or large spore subtypes), because the hyphae are present inside the hair.

It must be remembered that, sometimes, even human hair can be invaded in different ways. *T. violaceum*, e.g., can parasitize human hair by an endothrix or achorion mode of invasion. Animal hairs are often attacked in the same way as human hairs. Table 7 shows the known data. Photo 2 shows cattle hair invaded by *T. verrucosum* — the most common animal dermatophyte in Czechoslovakia.

XI. CULTIVATION

A prerequisite for establishing a diagnosis of veterinary dermatophytoses is the demonstration by cultivation of the causative agent. The main purpose of cultivation is to differentiate the causative agent from others causing similar dermatoses (e.g. skin diseases provoked by zooparasites, microbial dermatoses etc.). In this way a differential diagnosis may be made. The limited reliability of the results of microscopic examination of samples taken from cutaneous lesions of animals (see above) emphasizes that the cultivation must be performed consistently. Species differentiation, which is made possible by cultivation of the agent of the pathological process, assists in choosing suitable therapy, in estimating the course of the disease and its prognosis; this enables the attending veterinarian to make a more precise epizootological and epidemiological analysis (risk of contagion of other animals or man, way of spreading, necessity of safety precautions etc.). Cultivation is also the only method of conclusively revealing latent dermatophytoses or the carrying of dermatophytes by healthy animals as well as the existence of dermatophytes in extra-animal substrates, which may become primary sources of infection (soil, litter etc.).

For species identification it is necessary to isolate the dermatophyte from the lesion, to obtain a colony. Dermatophytes grow well on a wide range of cultivation media. However, the use of the glucose peptone agar medium known as Sabouraud's glucose agar, must be recommended because the behaviour of dermatophytes on this medium at 26 °C incubation temperature is well known. The macro- and micromorphological properties of colonies serve for identification. It must be noted that after several passages in vitro these properties may change remarkably.

a) Macromorphology of colonies

Dermatophytes can be identified on the basis of: rate of growth, ground plan, texture, surface colour, reverse colour.

1. Rate of growth

It seems that the rate of growth of a colony radius is one of the relatively constant properties of each dermatophyte so that the measurements of the

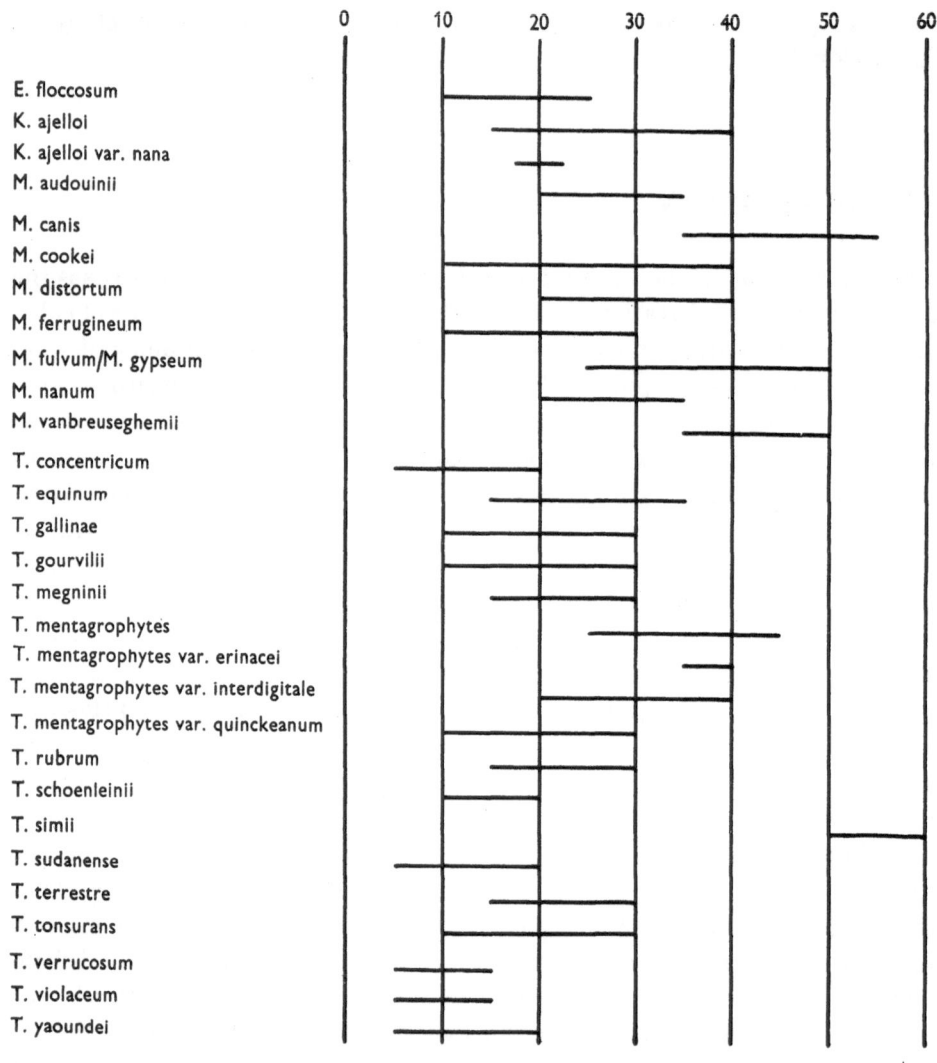

Fig. 8. Approximate diameter of colonies after 10 days (in mm).

colony diameter can be of value in the identification process. The radius or diameter of a colony increases in an approximately linear fashion under stable cultivation conditions. The rate of growth is dependent upon the medium used and on the incubation temperature. Fig. 8 shows the diameter of colonies growing on glucose peptone agar medium at 26 °C after 10 days. The data are in accord with our own observations and with those in the literature. There are clearly considerable differences among the individual strains isolated. Sometimes tubes, sometimes plates are used. The primary culture is often contaminated and a subculture must be made. Cultivation conditions are apt to vary considerably in different laboratories. It seems that the vast majority of dermatophytes grow better and more rapidly in subculture, but sometimes they grow even slower. In the light of these and other circumstances the given data can be only accepted as a general guide for the identification of dermatophytes in primary culture or in not too numerous (1—3) subcultures. Some dermatophytes grow relatively very rapidly — their colony diameter usually attains more than 40 mm at the end of 10 days (e.g. *M. canis, M. gypseum*). Others grow more slowly (e.g. *T. verrucosum* and *T. violaceum*) and their colonies measure not more than 15 mm in diameter. The colonies of *T. schoenleinii, T. sudanense, T. yaoundei, T. verrucosum* and *T. violaceum* grow very slowly especially in primary culture or the first subculture and can be considered to be "mature" after 20 days of incubation. *T. gallinae, E. floccosum, M. ferrugineum* are mature after about 15 days and the rest in about 10 days after inoculation. Maturity is the state when all important diagnostic properties are developed.

2. The ground plan

The surface of the colony (its aerial part, that part growing over the surface of the medium) develops in different stages. Table 8 shows the most frequently observed ground plans of individual dermatophytes. However, even this feature must be considered to be not always stable and Table 8 gives only an approximate indication.

3. The texture

Three main types of aerial colonies can be recognized macroscopically from their texture.

1. The membranous form (glabrous, waxy, humid, faviform): The aerial mycelium is entirely absent and the filamentous nature of the colony is,

with exception of the periphery, inapparent. The glabrous surface is due to the compact mass of vegetative mycelium which is prominent on the surface of the culture medium.

2. The filamentous form (cottony, fluffy, hairy, velvety, woolly): A more or less high and dense aerial mycelium is formed.
3. The granular-powdery form: Characterized by the absence of filamentous aerial elements.

The granulated surface texture is produced by the massive production of macroconidia and/or microconidia. Some dermatophytes produce abundant submerged mycelium, the aerial part of the colony is underdeveloped or practically absent. Table 9 shows the tendency of individual dermatophytes to form such textures. Sometimes, one part of the colony (e.g. the centre) is granular, another part (e.g. the margins) filamentous. Mixed or transient types are frequent. Table 10 demonstrates the tendency to form furrows and folds.

4. The surface colour

Table 11 gives the colours which can be observed on the surface of the colony after maturity. Sometimes, the colony is uniformly coloured, sometimes, there are various combinations of colours. Several dermatophyte species produce diffusible pigment, colouring the medium in the vicinity of the colony. In this work we have used PACLT's (1958) colour code and classification. The colour of the pigment produced depends on the pH of the medium. McGABE and MIER (1960) after studying the chemical composition of the pigment of *T. menta-grophytes*, *T. rubrum* and *T. violaceum* stated that it is of an anthrachinonous nature.

5. The reverse colour

Some dermatophytes are characterized by the reverse pigmentation of their colonies (e.g. *T. gallinae*, *T. megninii*). Sometimes, the reverse colour practically corresponds with the surface colour (e.g. in *E. floccosum*, *T. violaceum*). Table 8 lists the colours found on the reverse side of colonies.

6. Pleomorphic degeneration

In older parts of a granular or membranous colony (in its centre or almost in its centre), there sometimes appears a white, sterile, fluffy mycelium. This phenomenon is called pleomorphism or pleomorphic degeneration. *T. rubrum* mostly grows in a fluffy fashion so that its colony can be considered to be naturally pleomorphic. Some dermatophytes, which normally grow in a velvety form (e.g. *T. megninii*) can also be described as pleomorphic, whereby the sporulation is mostly remarkably reduced. While there is no sign of pleomorphism in the primary culture, the subculture may be atypically, completely pleomorphic. If the inoculum is taken from the pleomorphic part of the colony, it is highly probable that an entirely pleomorphic colony will appear in the subculture. The naturally pleomorphic species have been called "rubriform" by PALDROK (1953). By contrast "florentiform" species sporulate heavily. Central or paracentral fairly large areas can be observed even in relatively young primary cultures (e.g. in *E. floccosum, K. ajelloi, M. cookei, T. mentagrophytes*) which are granular, florentiform. We have repeatedly observed the formation of small pleomorphic tufts in typically membranous, glabrous colonies of *T. violaceum*. Our strains of *T. tonsurans*, grown typically for a long time, become entirely pleomorphic in subculture. The term pleomorphic degeneration seems to be incorrect (see HEJTMÁNEK 1964, WEITZMAN 1964).

7. Faviform degeneration

Sometimes, a fluffy *T. rubrum* colony forms a glabrous membranous zone. This phenomenon is called faviform degeneration. *T. violaceum*, e.g., grows from the beginning in membranous, glabrous colonies. Also here, this term seems to be incorrect. When the part on the surface of the medium is underdeveloped, a submerged type of growth is often observed in *T. verrucosum*.

However, even a typical colony of a species such as *M. cookei* starts to grow in submerged form in subculture without any obvious cause.

b) Micromorphology of colonies

The micromorphological properties of colonies can be examined by two methods. In slide culture or, if a normal colony is examined by the microscope, the elements remain in their natural position, but their shapes and structure cannot be viewed in detail. For precise studies, a microscopic preparation made from several parts taken from the radius of the colony (this will be explained later) must be used. However, this manipulation may deform the hyphae and liberate the spores.

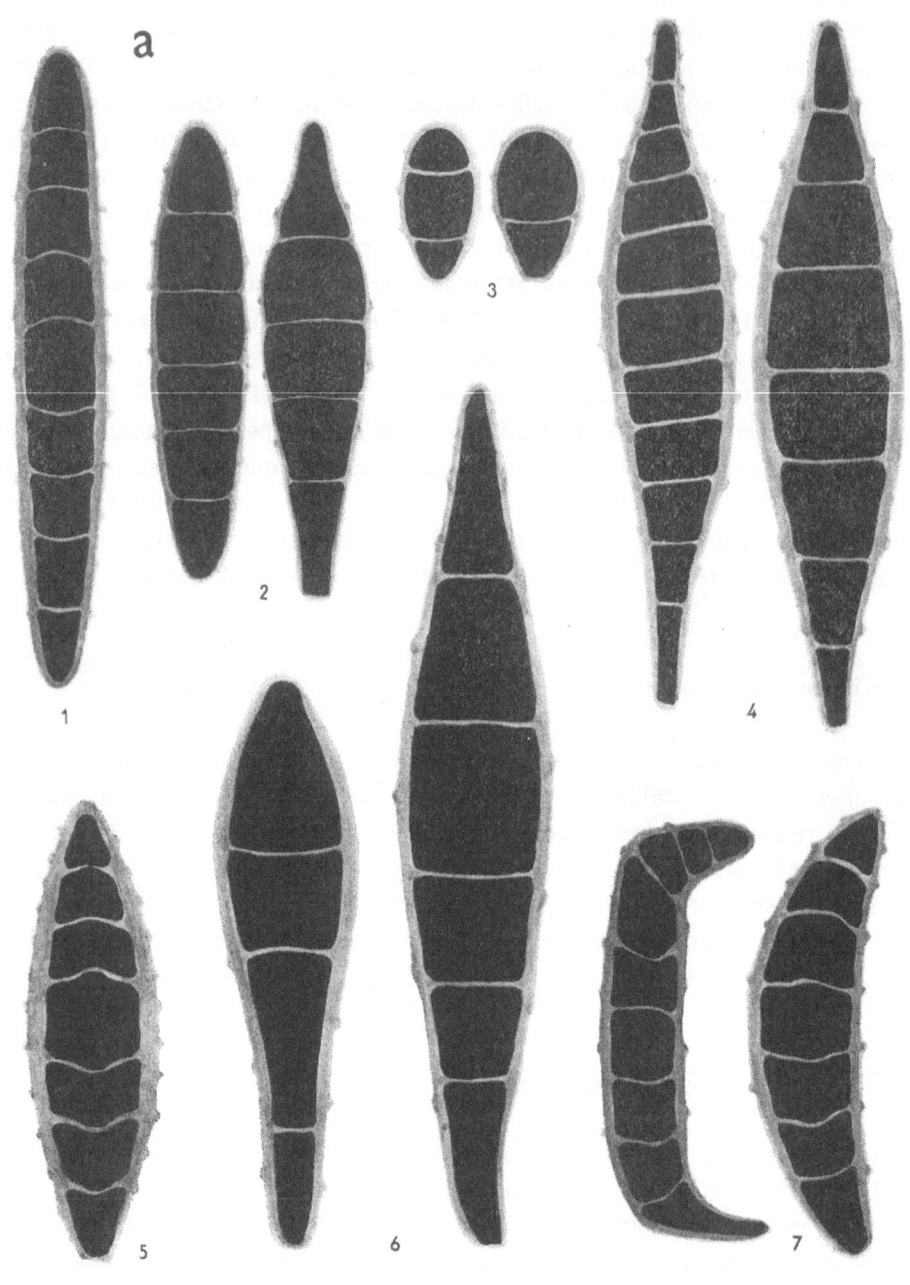

Fig. 9. Shape and structure of macroconidia observed (size not always typical).

a) 1 — *M. vanbreuseghemii*, 2 — *M. gypseum*, 3 — *M. nanum*, 4 — *M. canis*, 5 — *M. cookei*, 6 — *M. audouinii*, 7 — *M. distortum*.

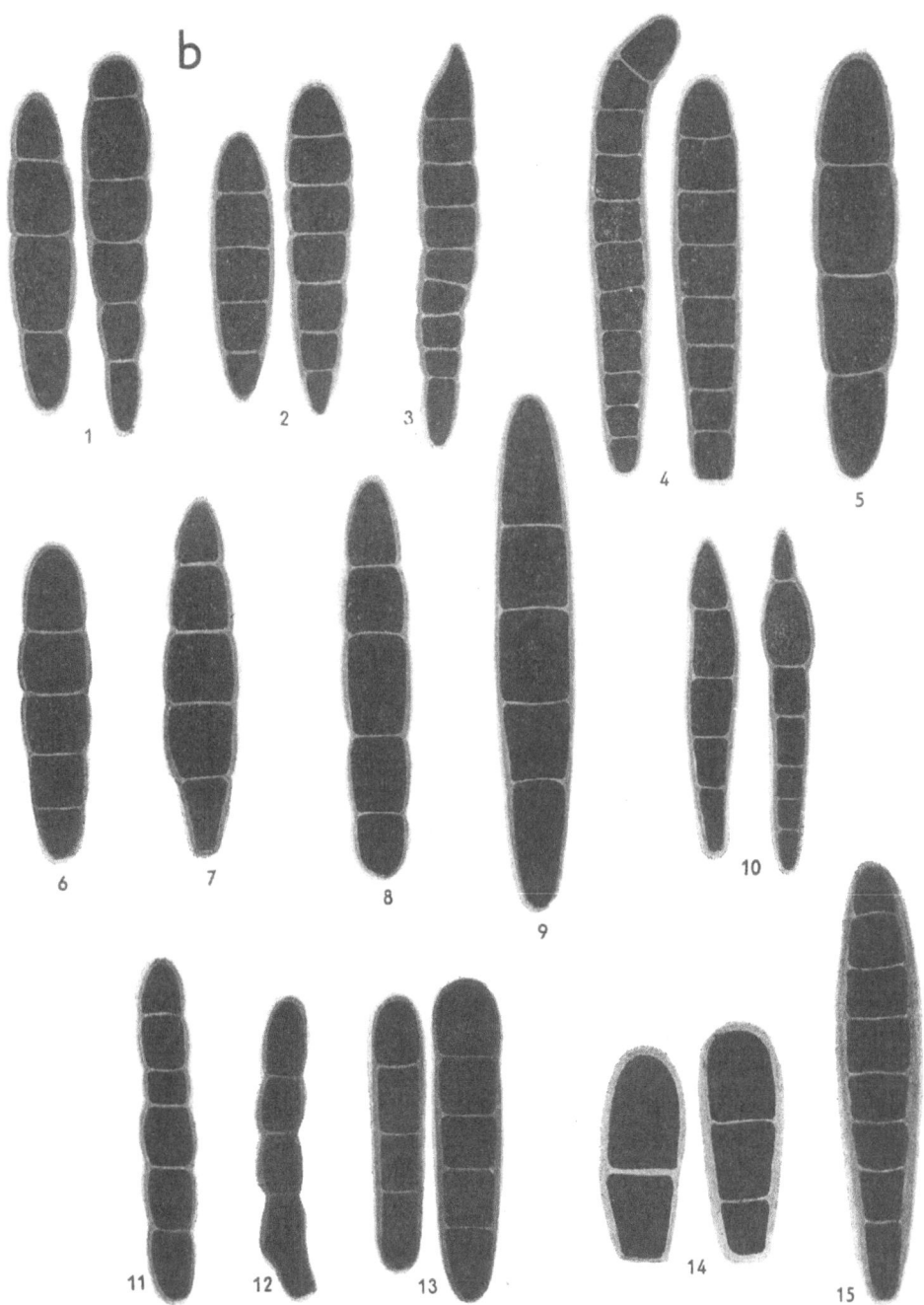

b) 1 — *T. mentagrophytes*, 2 — *T. mentagrophytes* var. *erinacei*, 3 — *T. mentagrophytes* var. *quinckeanum*, 4 — *T. rubrum*, 5 — *T. tonsurans*, 6 — *T. gallinae*, 7 — *T. equinum*, 8 — *T. megninii*, 9 — *T. simii*, 10 — *T. verrucosum*, 11 — *T. gourvilii*, 12 — *T. violaceum*, 13 — *T. terrestre* (typical), 14 — *E. floccosum*, 15 — *K. ajelloi* (typical).

8. Macroconidia

The most remarkable microscopic elements of dermatophytes are macroconidia (in French fuseaux, in German Spindeln). These reproductive elements may be numerous, rare or absent (e.g. *T. concentricum* does not produce these spores). If present, their shape and size can offer many valuable data for diagnosis. After studying the macroconidia of *M. cookei*, LENHART and HEJTMÁNEK (1963) made the following conclusions:

1. Significantly different average values of the size of macroconidia were obtained from different places in the same single spore colony.
2. The length and width of macroconidia, collected at the same distance from the centre of the colony after 12 and 41 days of cultivation, changed significantly.
3. The average length of macroconidia decreased significantly with the increasing distance from the centre of a 41 day-old colony.
4. The number of cells in the macroconidia depended likewise upon the age of the colony and the place from which the examined specimen of mycelium was taken.
5. The width of the macroconidia and the thickness of their membrane did not undergo such considerable changes as the number of cells during the ageing of the colony.
6. Evidence is given, in this paper, to confirm that it is necessary in the biometry of spores to adduce, in addition to cultivation conditions, also the age of the culture examined and the distance from the centre of the colony, at which the mycelium was collected.

The morphology of macroconidia (their shape and especially their structure) can also be influenced by the mounting fluid used (DVOŘÁK, HUBÁLEK and OTČENÁŠEK 1969). We recommend the use of iodine solution, which quickly kills these elements and makes them more distinct. It is necessary to examine such a preparation 10—30 minutes after its exposure to the iodine solution. In this time the changes in the structure of the macroconidia caused by iodine are completed. If saline is used, the macroconidia remain intact, but their structure cannot be satisfactorily distinguished. The cellular wall of the macroconidia seems to thicken after a 10 min exposure to iodine, but these changes seem to be constant and, therefore, the use of iodine solution may be permitted although even artificial values may be obtained.

Table 13 shows the number of macroconidia produced by the individual dermatophytes. The given data were mostly obtained from the study of older and mature colonies.

Fig. 9 shows the shape and structure of macroconidia found by us in dermatophytic colonies. Firstly, the shape of macroconidia will be briefly discussed.

Macroconidia can be straight or bent. Bent macroconidia are frequently found in colonies of *M. distortum* and *M. vanbreuseghemii*. The following basic shapes of macroconidia may be distinguished: egg-shaped, pear-shaped, club-shaped, spindle-shaped, short and thick with rounded ends, relatively long and thin with pointed ends.

Table 14 shows the shapes of macroconidia, observed in the individual dermatophyte species, Fig. 10 the number or macroconidial cells and Table 15 the size of macroconidia.

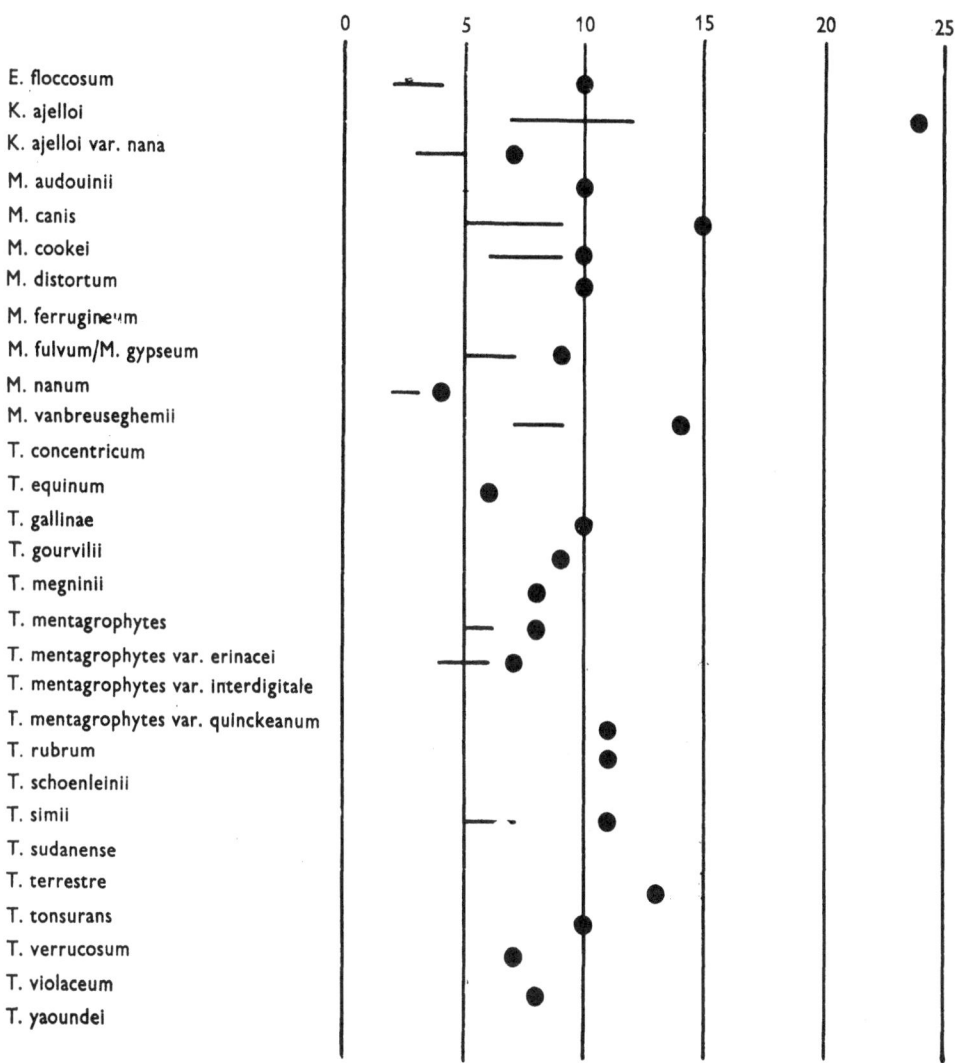

Fig. 10. Number of macroconidial "cells" (● maximal number observed, ——— most frequent number of "cells").

9. Microconidia (aleuries, aleuriospores)

The second fructification element of a dermatophytic colony are the micro-conidia. They also can be numerous, rare or absent. E.g. they are not produced by *E. floccosum* and *T. schoenleinii* (Table 16). The morphology of microconidia does not usually supply satisfactorily reliable data for diagnostic purposes.

10. Modes of conidial production

Macroconidia and microconidia are the spores of aerial mycelium produced in various ways. Both principally develop from the sides or the tips of the hyphae (Fig. 11, 12).

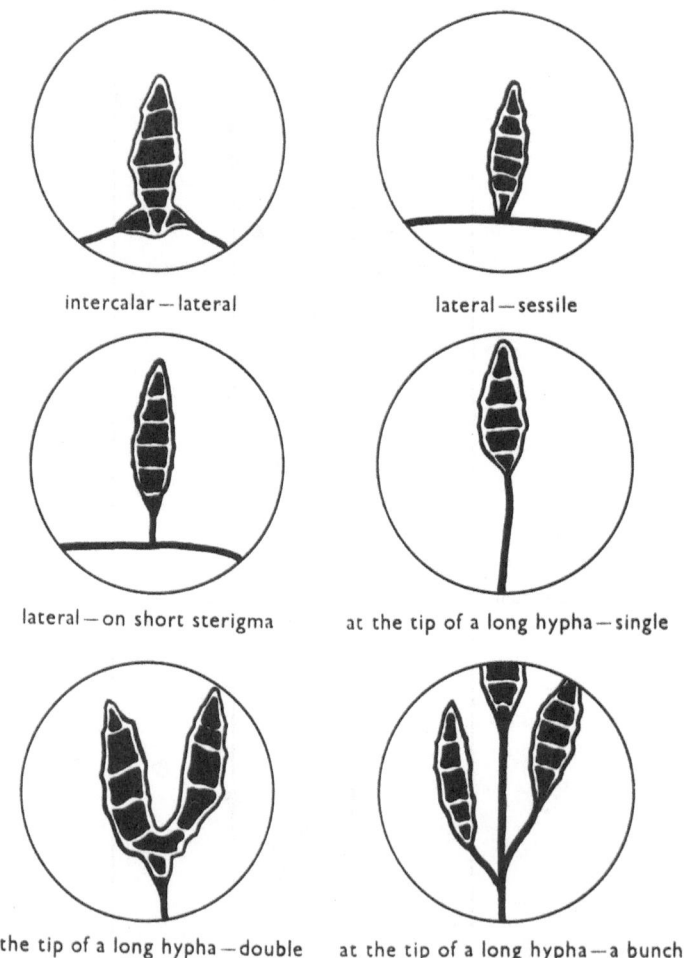

intercalar — lateral   lateral — sessile

lateral — on short sterigma   at the tip of a long hypha — single

at the tip of a long hypha — double   at the tip of a long hypha — a bunch

Fig. 11. Modes of macroconidia formation in *M. canis.*

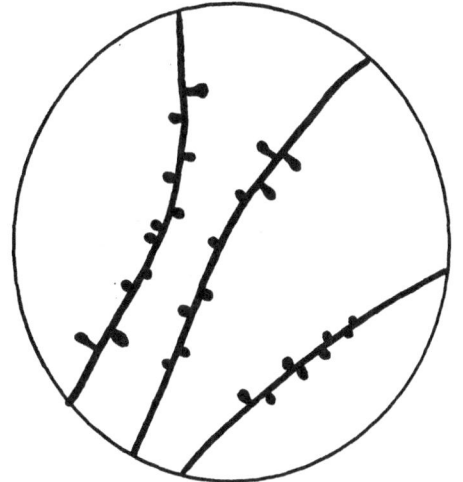

Simple sporiferous hyphae, acladium type of microconidia
formation ("en thyrse")

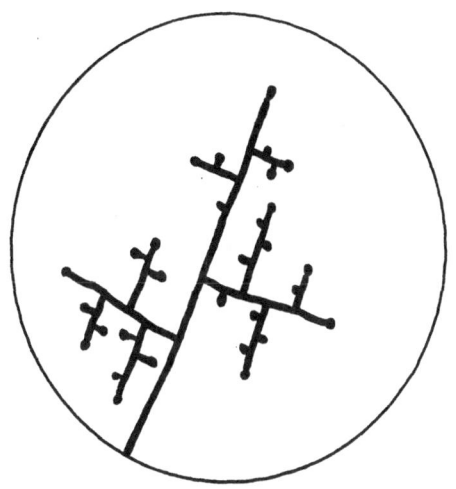

Botrytis type of microconidia formation ("en grappe")

Fig. 12. Modes of microconidia formation.

11. Germination of conidia and mycelium formation

Macroconidia and microconidia germinate under suitable conditions. One or
more germ tubes develop in a relatively short time (Fig. 13). The hyphae
grow, branch and anastomose.

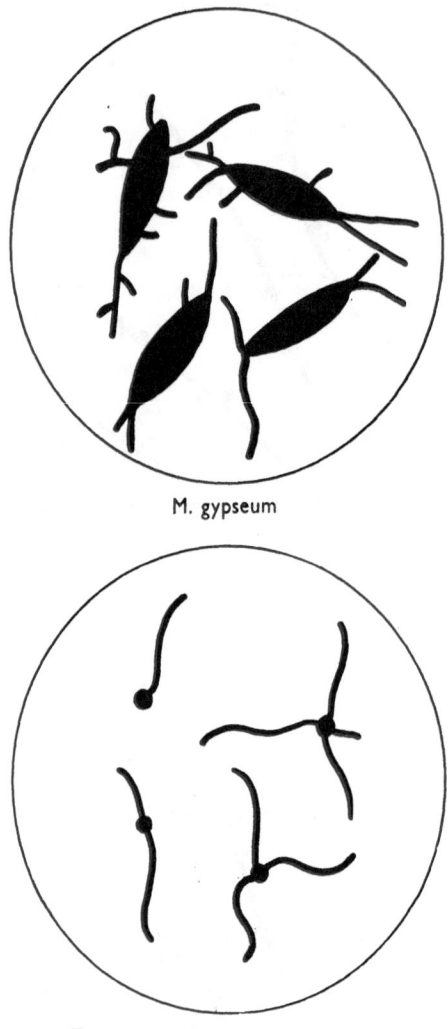

M. gypseum

T. mentagrophytes var. interdigitale

Fig. 13. Modes of macroconidial and micro-
conidial germination.

The structure of the mycelium

At the present, the structure of the mycelium cannot be used as a reliable means of diagnosis. A further special type of branching is the formation of elements known as pectinate hyphae (in French-organes pectinés, in German-kammzinkenförmiges Myzel). Several dermatophytes such as *M. ferrugineum* and *T. tonsurans* normally produce these elements. The so-called favic chandeliers (in German-kronleuchterartiges Myzel) are practically always present in the colonies of *M. distortum*, *M. ferrugineum*, *T. concentricum*, *T. schoenleinii*, *T. verrucosum* and *T. violaceum*. Especially *T. mentagrophytes* forms the so-called spirals (coils) (in French — spires, vrilles, in German — Weinranken), which are more or less contorted hyphae. Nodular bodies (in French-organes nodulaires, in German — knotenförmiges Myzel) are occasionally present in colonies of various dermatophytes. *M. ferrugineum, T. concentricum, T. megni-nii, T. schoenleinii, T. tonsurans, T. verrucosum, T. violaceum* do not produce them. The last elements which merit attention are racquet hyphae (hyphal cells with enlarged ends). They occur with variable frequency in the colonies of practically all dermatophytes. Fig. 14 shows all these special hyphal struc-tures. Practically all dermatophytes are capable of bearing in vitro chlamydo-spores and arthrospores (see Fig. 15).

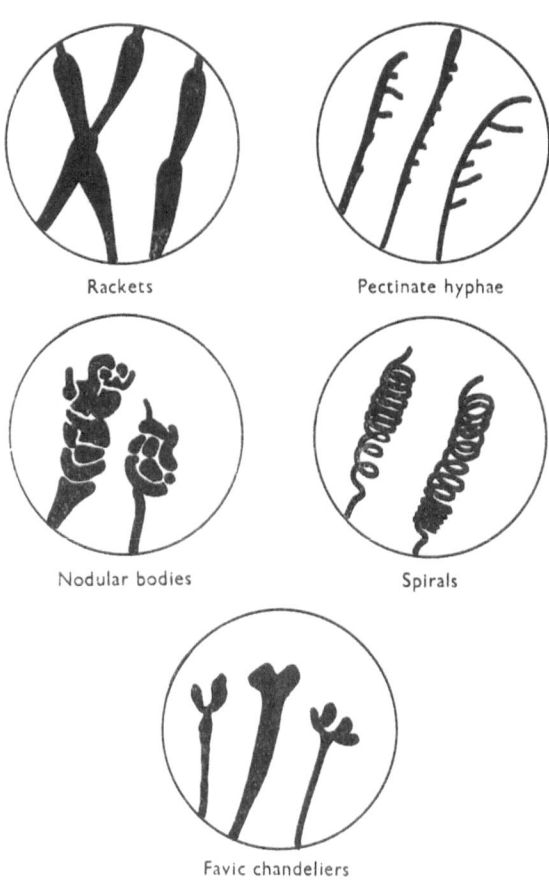

Rackets

Pectinate hyphae

Nodular bodies

Spirals

Favic chandeliers

Fig. 14. Special hyphal formations.

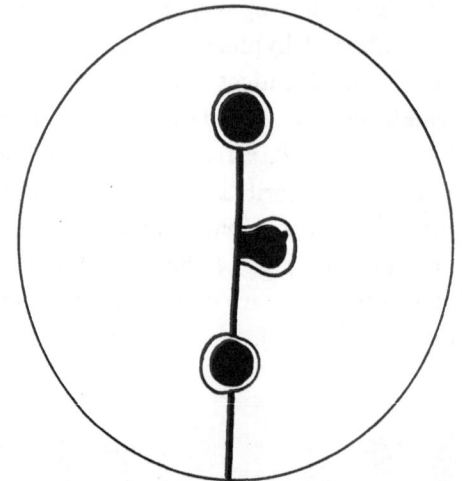

Chlamydospores (terminal, lateral, intercalar position)

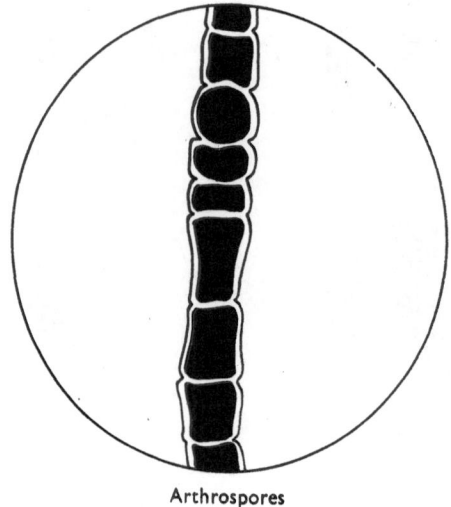

Arthrospores

Fig. 15. Spores of vegetative mycelium.

Micromorphology of the colonies is presented on the Photos 3 – 13.

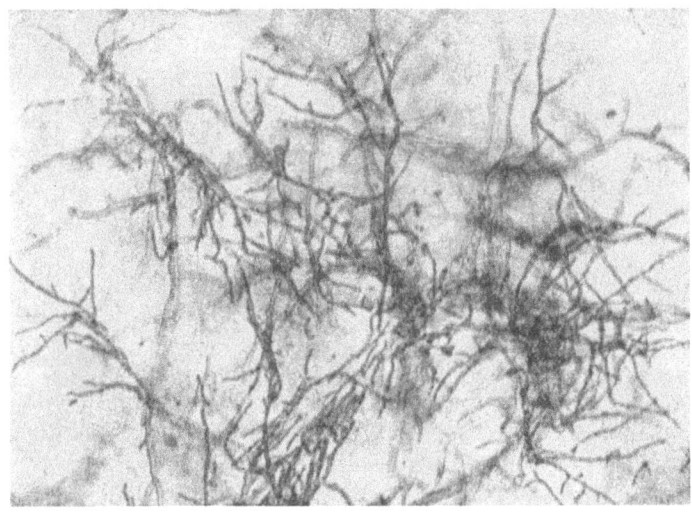

Phot. 3. Mycelium of *T. violaceum*, iodine solution after 10 min.
(approx. × 250).

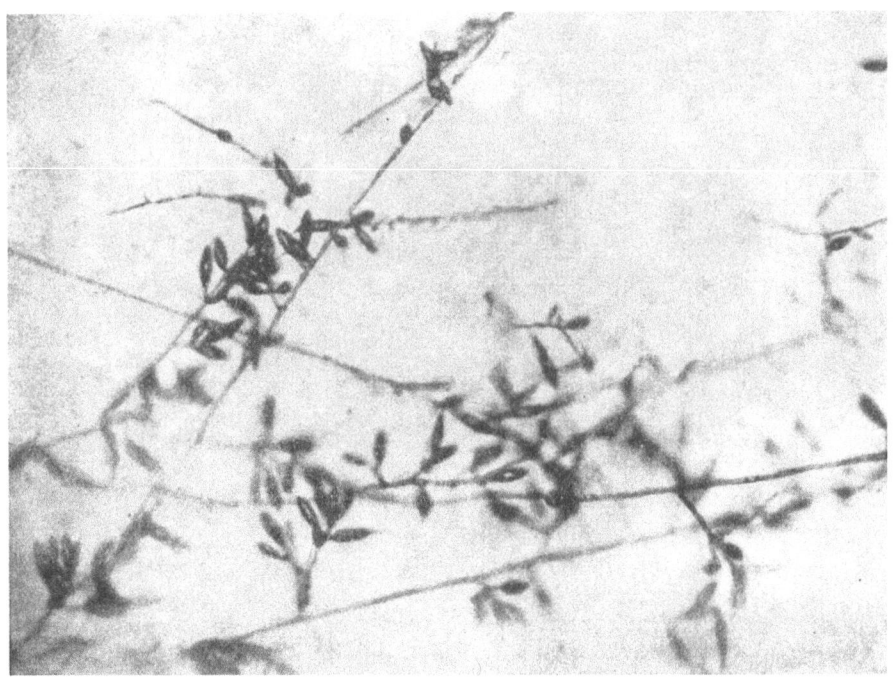

Phot. 4. Mycelium with macroconidia of *M. gypseum*; slide culture (approx. × 100).

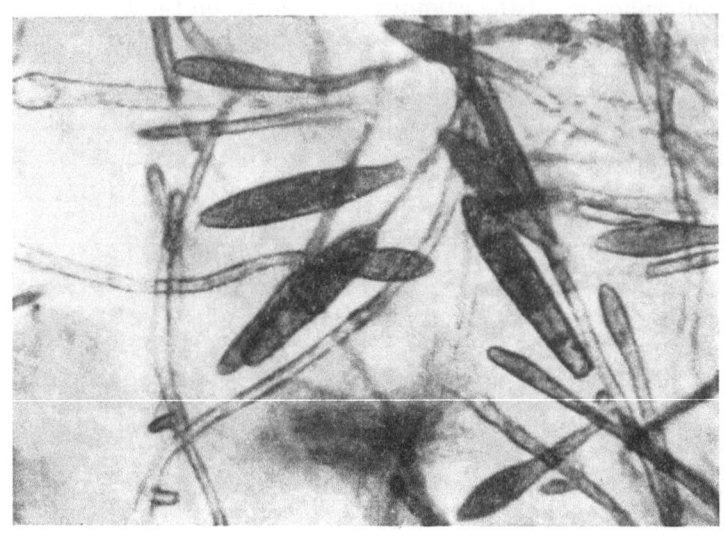

Phot. 5. Young macroconidia of *M. gypseum*; iodine solution after 10 min (approx. × 750).

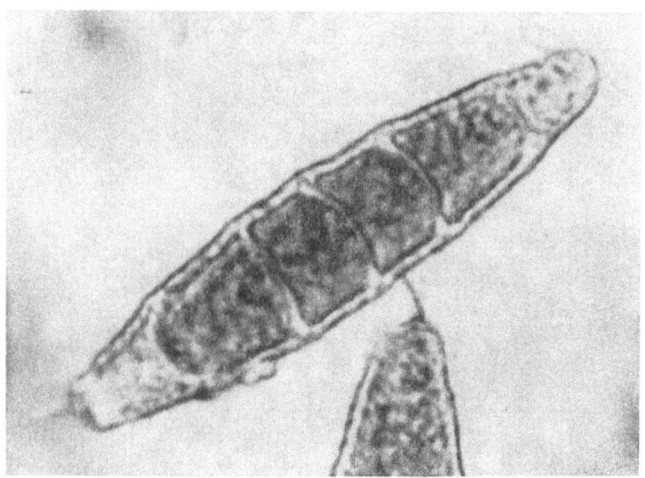

Phot. 6. Mature macroconidium of *M. gypseum*; iodine solution after 10 min (approx. × 200).

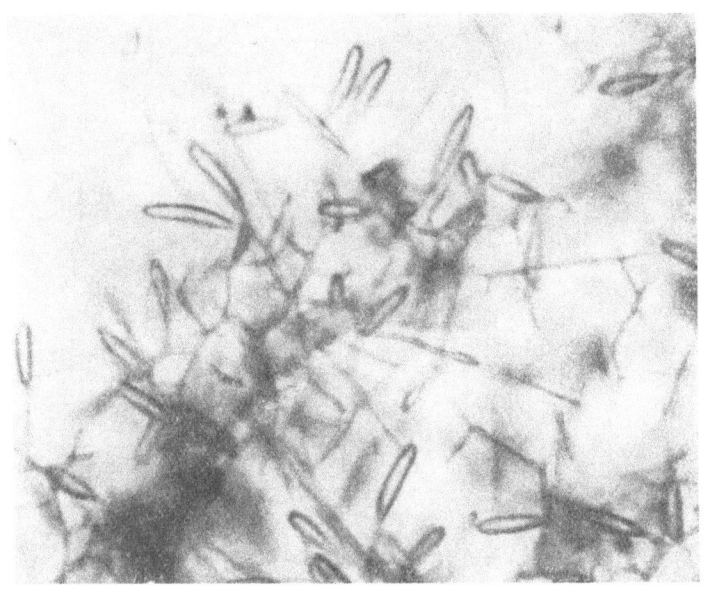

Phot. 7. Mycelium with macroconidia of *K. ajelloi*; slide culture (approx. × 275).

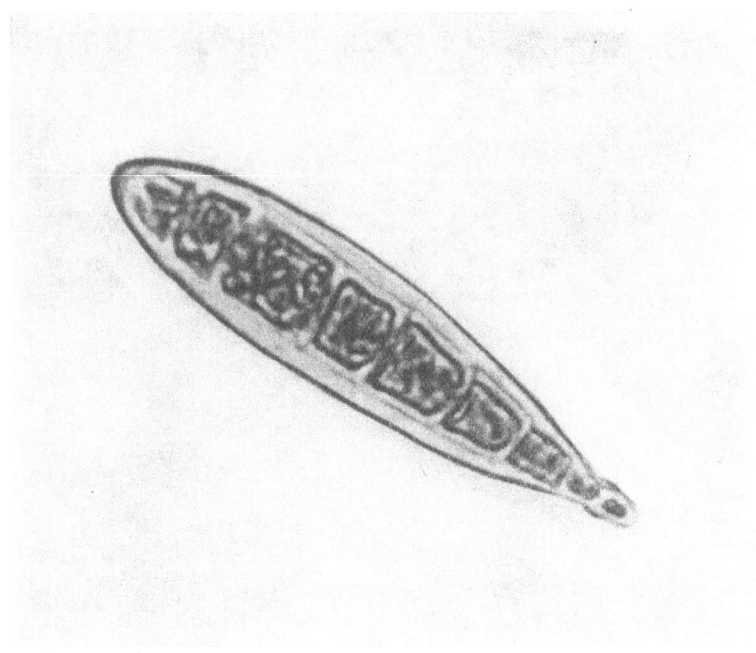

Phot. 8. Mature macroconidium of *K. ajelloi*; iodine solution after 10 min (× 2,000).

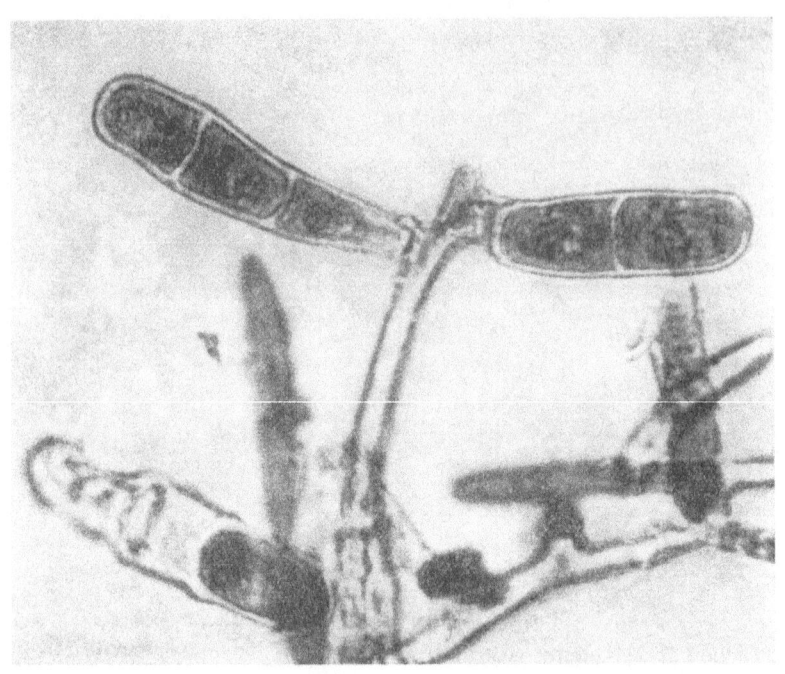

Phot. 9. Sessile macroconidia of *E. floccosum*; iodine solution after
10 min (× 1,500).

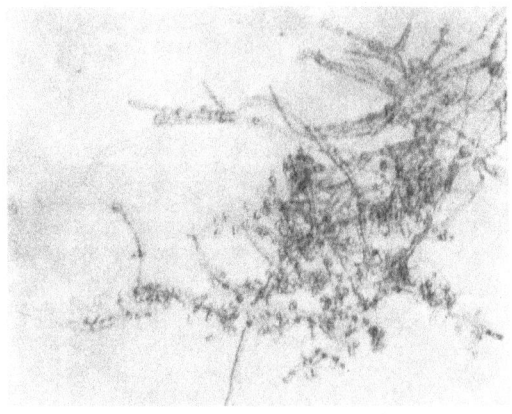

Phot. 10. Microconidia of *T. tonsurans*; iodine
solution after 10 min (approx. × 250).

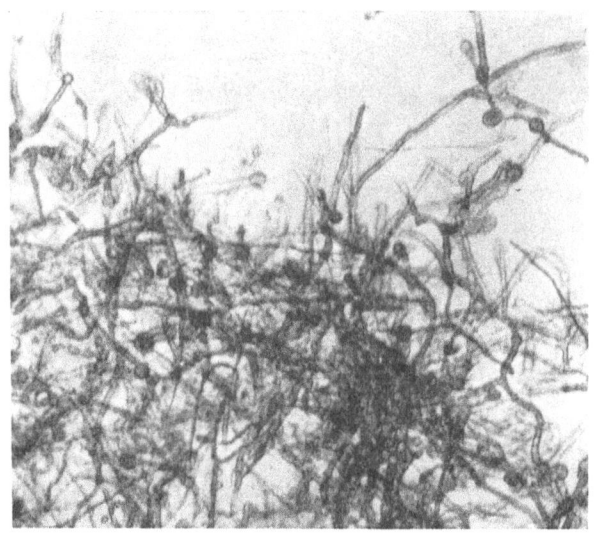

Phot. 11. Chlamydospores of *T. tonsurans*; iodine solution
after 10 min (approx. × 250).

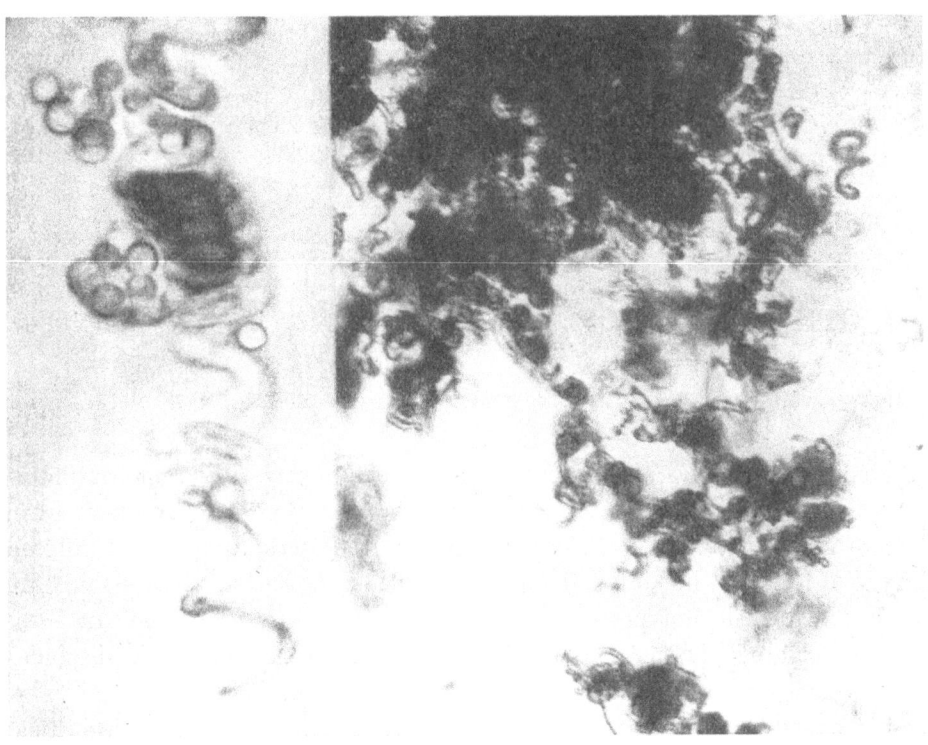

Phot. 12. Spirals of *T. mentagrophytes*; iodine solution after 10 min (approx. × 1,000,
approx. × 300).

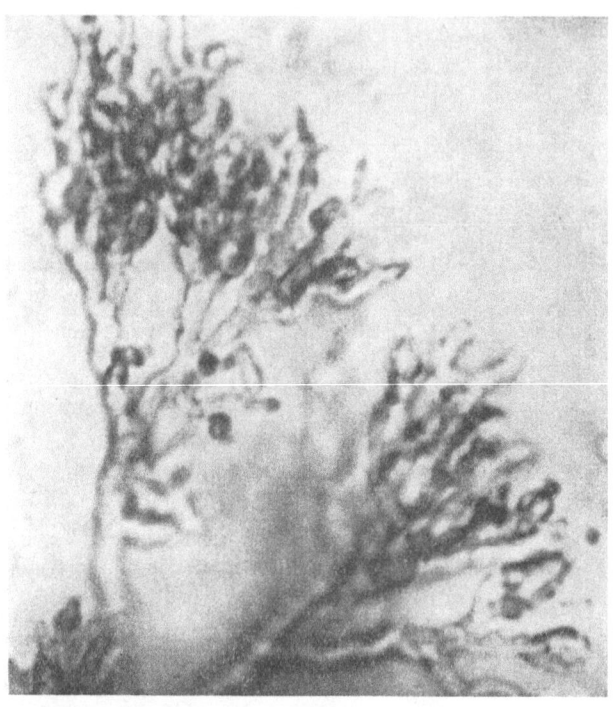

Phot. 13. Favic chandeliers of *T. verrucosum*; iodine
solution after 10 min (approx. × 500).

XII. OTHER METHODS

1. Differential diagnosis

Macromorphologically and micromorphologically very different dermatophytes such as *E. floccosum* and *T. mentagrophytes* cannot be confused even
if the strains isolated are not entirely typical. Other dermatophytes, if isolated
in typical form, do not offer diagnostic problems. However, often strains are
obtained which do not possess all important diagnostic properties. In these
cases, other auxiliary methods must be used. Sometimes, the strain becomes
more typical after reisolation. The result of inoculation itself can be of value
for identification. The hair keratinolysis in vitro, the induction of fructifications cleistothecia or macroconidia formation, biochemical tests, the observation
of older cultures or of subcultures may sometimes be very helpful in identification. Fig. 16 shows the most commonly occurring diagnostic problems.

Sometimes, if atypical intermediary (transient) strains are isolated, the experimental inoculation of animals can be of valuable diagnostic aid. In general, anthropophilic dermatophytes are nonpathogenic, while zoophilic strains are pathogenic as would be expected. We recommend the intracutaneous inoculation of guinea-pigs for the diagnosis (see C VIII). Sometimes, the clinical aspect of the lesion or the way the hair is invaded, offers valuable data.

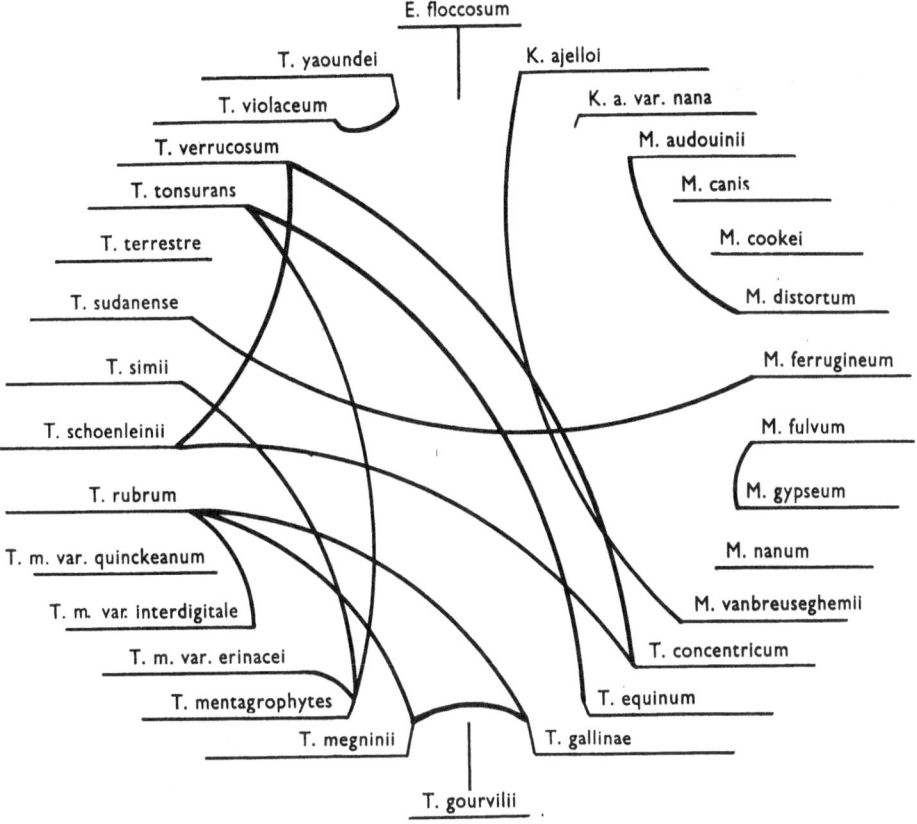

Fig. 16. Differential diagnosis.

In general, the results of inoculation are dependent on the strain examined. Freshly isolated, abundantly sporulating strains from animals easily produce lesions. The inoculation procedure is very important for a successful development of the lesion.

2. Animal inoculation

Animal inoculation plays only an auxiliary role in the diagnosis because susceptibility or resistance of the animal cannot be estimated and defined.

Data from the literature on the results of animal inoculations are often not convincing; sometimes only a few strains could be examined so that the survey reported in Table 17 cannot offer a fully reliable picture of the results of guinea-pig inoculations. It must be appreciated that the results of our experiments are concerned only with dermatophytes isolated in Czechoslovakia.

3. Keratinolysis of hairs in vitro

Keratinolysis of hairs in vitro has been studied by many authors (e.g. PARTRIDGE 1959, ZIEGLER and BÖHME 1963, FRIEDRICH 1964). Some differences have been observed to occur among different dermatophytes so that it may be possible to use this method as a diagnostic aid. THURNER (1966), using hairs of various animals (cattle, dog, goat, guinea-pig, horse, mouse) and of man, studied the ways, in which keratinolysis occurs with several dermatophytes. She observed that, in general, the hairs can be d sintegrated in two ways:

a) rectangular to the axis of the hair,
b) coaxial.

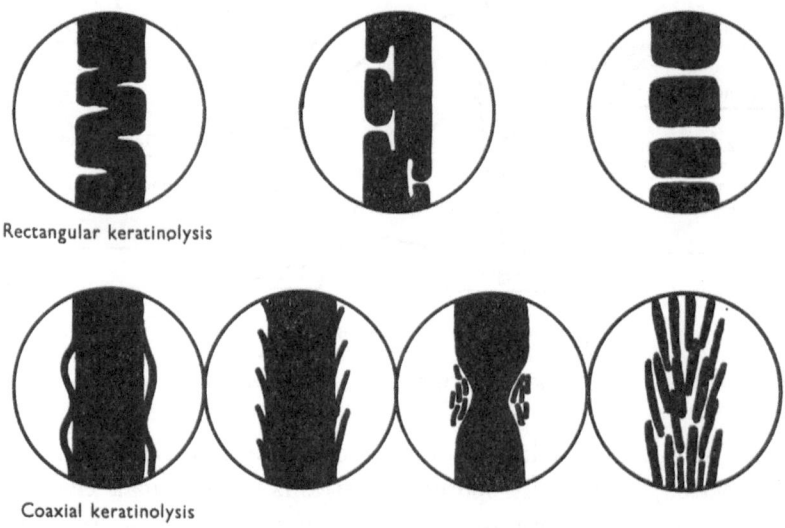

Rectangular keratinolysis

Coaxial keratinolysis

Fig. 17. Modes of hair keratinolysis in vitro.

For description of the method see chapter C VII 3. The ways of keratinolysis are schematically demonstrated in Fig. 17. Table 18 shows the various ways of keratinolysis as demonstrated on the hairs of the mammals in question. The hairs of guinea-pigs are attacked coaxially by all dermatophytes so that

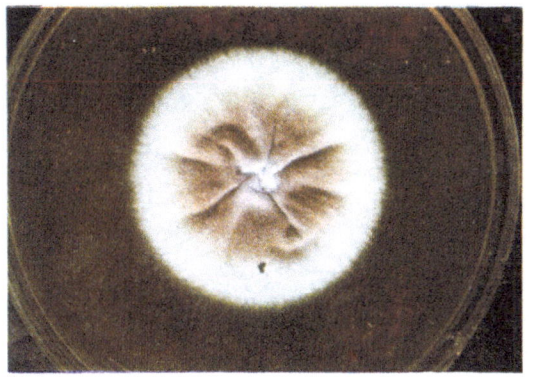

1. *Microsporon cookei* (5·2 cm)

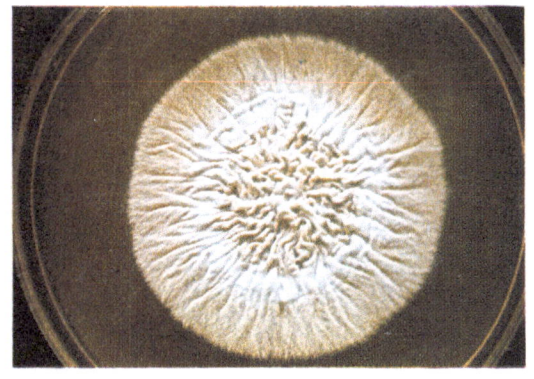

2. *M. ferrugineum* (6·0 cm)

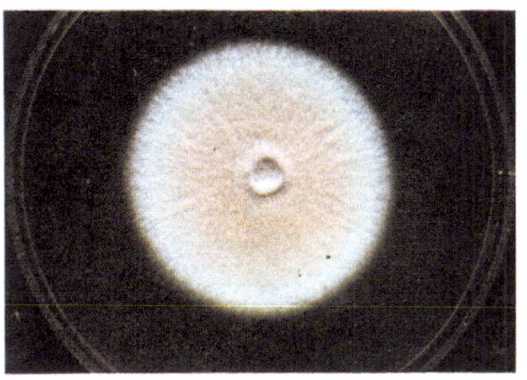

3. *M. gypseum* (7·3 cm)

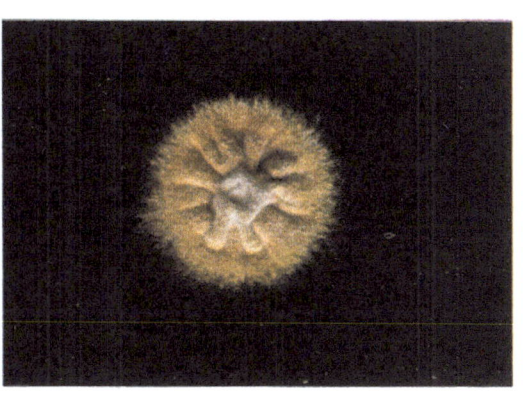

4. *M. nanum* (2·4 cm)

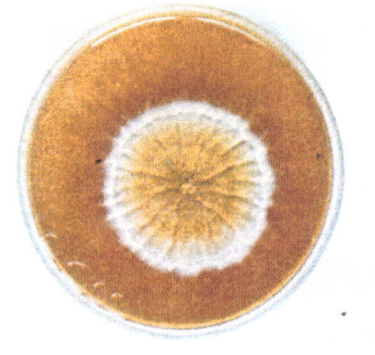

5. *M. vanbreuseghemii* (5·1 cm)

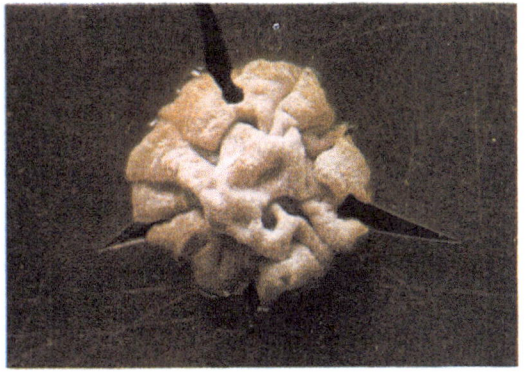

6. *Trichophyton concentricum* (1·3 cm)

(Real diameters in brackets)

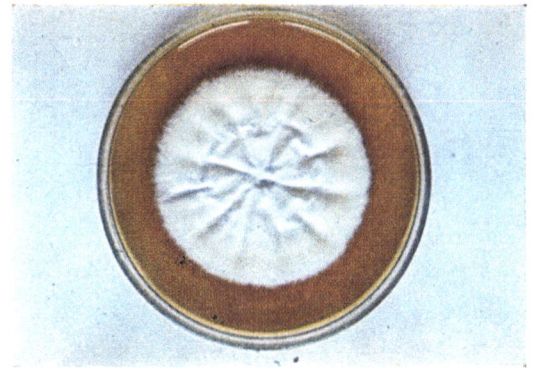

7. *T. equinum* (7·5 cm)

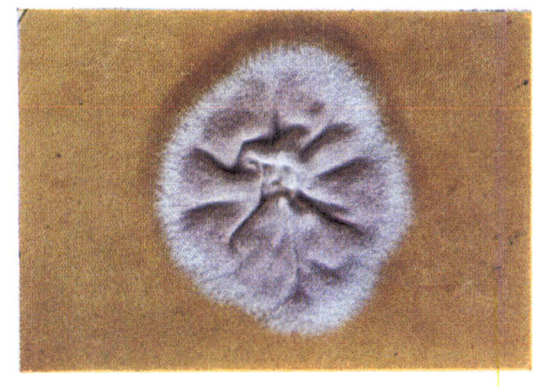

8. *T. megninii* (3·9 cm)

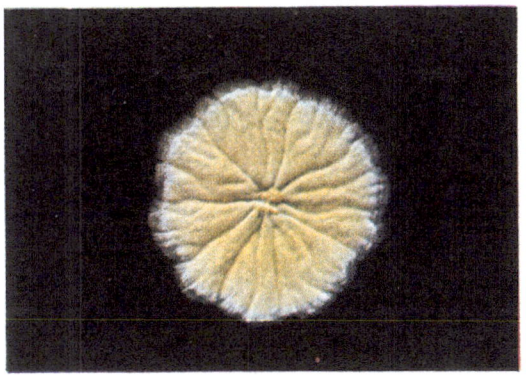

9. *T. sudanense* (3·1 cm)

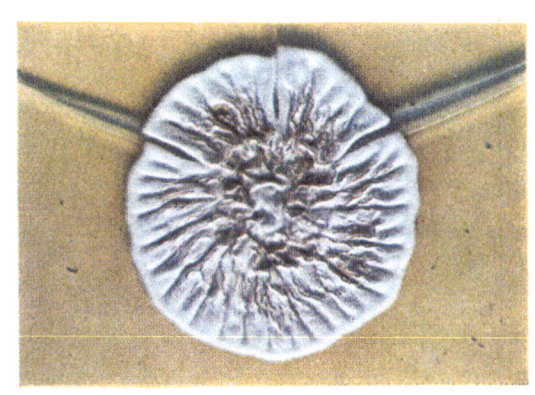

10. *T. tonsurans* (3·9 cm)

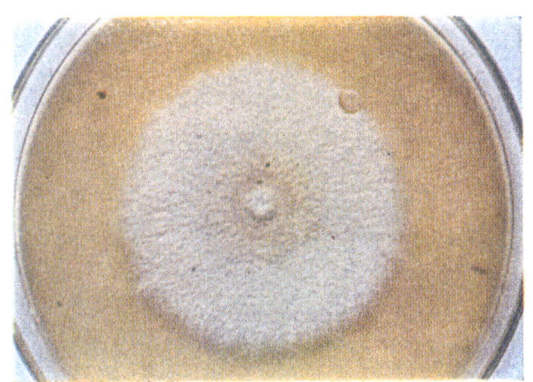

11. *T. vanbreuseghemii* (5·5 cm)

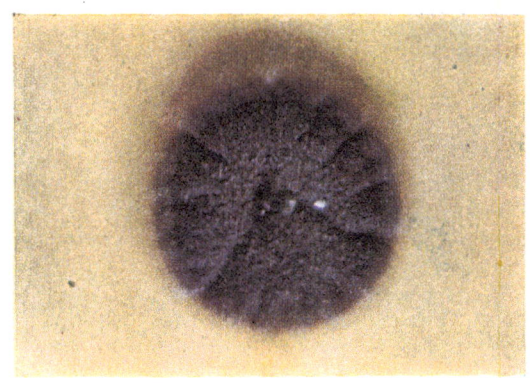

12. *T. violaceum* (1·4 cm)

this helps in identification. No differences exist between *T. mentagrophytes* and *T. m.* var. *interdigitale* and between *T. terrestre* and *T. verrucosum*.

As evident from the Table, hairs are frequently d'sintegrated by both coaxial and rectangular keratinolysis or they may remain intact. The method must be considered as supplementary and its diagnostic value must be verified.

4. Nutritional tests

AJELLO et al. (1963) summarized the nutritional patterns of some *Trichophyton* species. It has been shown that it may be possible to use these tests for identification (Table 19).

5. Perfect states

Some dermatophytes have corresponding perfect states. (For details see e.g. KUNERT and OTČENÁŠEK 1968.) The conditions for the production of cleisto-

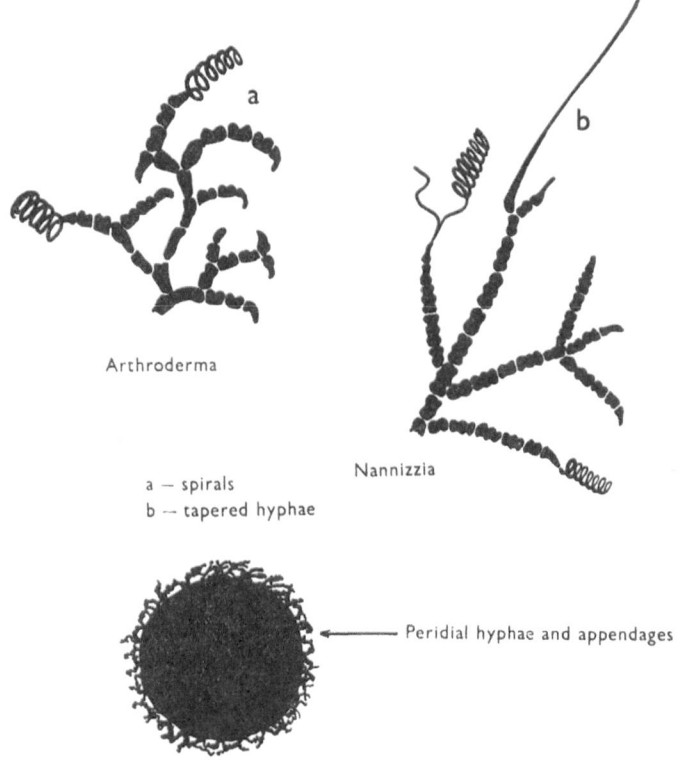

Fig. 18. Perfect states of *Arthroderma* and *Nannizzia*. Peridial hyphae and appendages.

thecia, for the transformation of imperfect forms to perfect forms are described elsewhere (see C IX). Fig. 18 and the survey reported in Table 20 and 21 show the most important characteristics of *Arthroderma* and *Nannizzia* species, which have their imperfect forms among dermatophytes.

B. SPECIAL ASPECTS

Zoophilic dermatophytes rarely attacking man

Many problems appear when descriptions are given of dermatophytes such as *T. equinum* and *T. gallinae*. Unfortunately, reports concerning these dermatophytes are relatively scarce in recent world literature. Our studies of *T. equinum* were conducted on several strains isolated from an epizootic outbreak identified by us, and on strains obtained from human lesions. *T. gallinae* we have so far isolated only once from a human lesion. We have studied numerous strains of these dermatophytes from various parts of the world, but some of them we found not entirely typical after repeated passages (in subculture).

Trichophyton equinum (Matruchot et Dassonville) Gedoelst, 1902

Perfect state: not known.

Discovered in 1898. Some authors considered it to be identical with *T. mentagrophytes* (CONANT et al. 1955, FRÁGNER 1958 a. o.). At the International Congress of Dermatology in Stockholm (1957) GEORG submitted a system including *T. equinum* as a valid species. The confusion with other dermatophytes (e.g. *T. mentagrophytes* and *T. tonsurans*) may be expected and the knowledge of these dermatophytes is far from complete. *T. equinum* is not identical with *Microsporon equinum* Guéguen, 1904.

Distribution

Saprophytic habitat and source of infection is not known. Causes dermatophytoses of horses (especially young horses), infections of man are rare and transmitted always from the horse. These dermatophytes occur during epizootic outbreaks among horsemen (BUCHVALD and VALENTOVÁ 1965) and among horsekeepers (OTČENÁŠEK et al. 1964). We have no knowledge of reliable reports of infection of animals other than horses. *T. equinum* seems to be a dermatophyte highly specialized for parasitic life on the horse. Recently, dermatophytoses of horses or man caused by this dermatophyte have been reported from America (BATTE and MILLER 1953, GEORG, KAPLAN and LA VERNE 1957, KRAL and SCHWARTZMANN 1964), Canada (BLANK and EREAUX 1964), from Brasil (LONDERO, FISCHMAN and RAMOS 1964), Australia (CONNOLE 1963), Great Britain (AINSWORTH and AUSTWICK 1955, GENTLES and O'SULLIVAN 1957, ENGLISH 1961), Germany (PETZOLD, RIETH and MERKT 1965), Yugoslavia (OŽEGOVIĆ and GRIN 1963), Czechoslovakia (OTČENÁŠEK, DVOŘÁK and SOVA 1962, BUCHVALD 1964). It probably occurred also in Bulgaria and the U.S.S.R. (COUDERT 1964). This dermatophyte seems to be distributed all over the world. In the U.S.A. it is the commonest cause of equine ringworm (GEORG, KAPLAN and CAMP 1957).

Brief characteristics of the disease

Lesions occur on the head (forehead, cheeks), on the neck, withers (in race-horses in the region of the saddle), the posterior area of the rump, the ventral area of the chest. They are oval or irregular in shape. Pathogenic changes are at first marked by loss of hair. The hairless skin is generally not inflamed, but covered with minute scales. Sometimes blisters are formed, which burst later and form crusts. These changes are accompanied by severe itching (KRAL 1964). The foci may become confluent, but are never covered with crusts as distinctly as in cattle (AINSWORTH and AUSTWICK 1959).

In experimentally infected horses the skin becomes edematous and lamellar crusts are formed after an incubation period of 3—6 days. The thickened skin becomes slightly furrowed. Hairs can easily be pulled out and are shed after 3—4 weeks (JAKSCH 1963). Young horses are more susceptible than are older horses (CONNOLE 1963, KRAL 1964).

Diseases of horses observed by us may be clinically characterized as herpes tonsurans maculosus or herpes tonsurans vesiculosus (OTČENÁŠEK, DVOŘÁK and SOVA 1962). This applies also to the diseases observed in Slovakia (BUCHVALD 1964).

In man, *T. equinum* may cause tinea capitis, tinea barbae or tinea corporis. No fluorescence of infected hairs.

Direct microscopy

Hair invasion of the endoectothrix type with large extrapilar spores (3·5—8 μm). In the skin scales, branched, septate more or less arthrosporulated hyphae are found.

Colony macromorphology

The colony diameter attains 15—35 mm at the end of 10 days. The ground plan of the mature colony is mostly regular — circular to slightly asteroid.

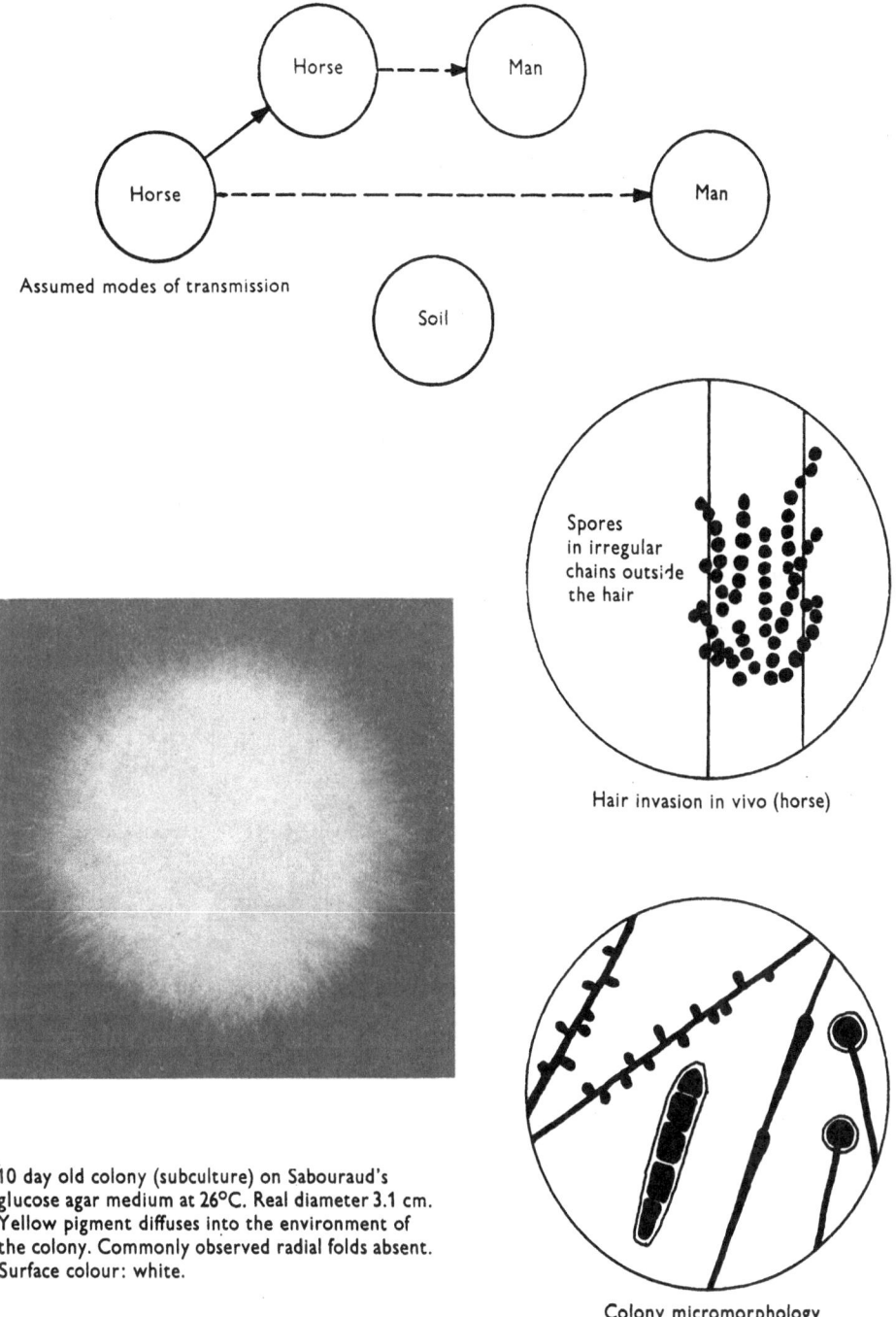

Assumed modes of transmission

Spores
in irregular
chains outside
the hair

Hair invasion in vivo (horse)

10 day old colony (subculture) on Sabouraud's
glucose agar medium at 26°C. Real diameter 3.1 cm.
Yellow pigment diffuses into the environment of
the colony. Commonly observed radial folds absent.
Surface colour: white.

Colony micromorphology

Fig. 19. *Trichophyton equinum* (Matruchot et Dassonville) Gedoelst 1902. World
wide registered dermatophyte, attacking mainly horses.

The surface is velvety to velvety powdered, in some strains entirely flat. Other strains form an umbilicus in the centre, which may be either elevated or depressed. Some irregular radial furrows develop in the paracentral zone. The periphery is flat, covering the agar surface. At first, the surface is white with a bright yellow pigment in the periphery. Its colour may also be pale rose or salmon. Later, the surface becomes cream to tan coloured. The diffusible pigment of our strains are a pale lemon yellow, lemon yellow to yellow. At first, the reverse side is a bright yellow, then pink to deep reddish brown. It may also be saffron yellow to orange. The pigment diffuses occasionally remarkably into the medium developing a peripheral ring.

Colony micromorphology

The branched septate hyphae measure $2-3\cdot5$ μm in diameter. Macroconidia may be absent or are almost always present in limited numbers only. They are clavate to cigar-shaped, smooth, with thin walls, $2-6$ cells, size $4-12$ by $10-67$ μm. Microconidia are always found either in low or large numbers. They are ovoid, clavate to pyriform and measure $1-4$ by $2-5$ μm. Mostly, they develop directly from the sides (or on short sterigmata) of simple, sporiferous hyphae (acladium type). Our strains formed racquets and chlamydospores.

Differential diagnosis

Sometimes, *T. equinum* must be differentiated from *T. mentagrophytes* or *T. tonsurans*.

Experimental pathogenicity

The cultures are always pathogenic for guinea-pigs and rabbits. An erythematosquamous lesion measuring $2-3$ cm develops after 10 days. Sometimes, typical endoectothrix invasion of hair of the large spore subtype can be observed. The lesions regularly heal without treatment after 30 days.

Keratinolysis of hairs in vitro

T. equinum does not attack the hairs of goat, man and mouse. On the long axis, rectangular keratinolysis has been observed on the hairs of dogs, coaxial keratinolysis on the hairs of cattle and both rectangular and coaxial keratinolysis on the hairs of horses.

Nutritional requirements

T. equinum does not grow on vitamine free media. All strains need nicotinic acid.

64

Trichophyton gallinae (Mégnin) Silva et Benham, 1952

Perfect state: not known.

Synonyms: *Epidermophyton gallinae* Mégnin, 1881; *Achorion gallinae* Sabouraud, 1910; *Sabouraudites gallinae* Ota et Langeron, 1923; *Microsporum gallinae* Grigorakis, 1929.

Some authors considered it to be identical with *T. megninii* (CONANT et al. 1954 a.o.). SILVA and BENHAM (1952) have shown that it must be separated as a valid species, which can be clearly differentiated from *T. megninii*.

Distribution

Saprophytic habitat and course of infection not known. This species seems to be highly specialized for parasitic life on gallinaceous birds. It causes mainly dermatophytoses in chickens (attacking more often cocks than hens) and turkeys. Infection of other birds seems to be rare (canary — KRAL 1962, black grouse — PÄTIÄLÄ 1951, pigeon — GIERLOFF and KATIČ 1961). Occasional dermatophytoses of other animals caused by this dermatophyte have also been reported: dog and mouse (GIERLOFF and KATIČ 1961), cat (BÜHLMAN and RIETH 1962). Human cases are likewise exceptional (e.g. ROSETTI 1942, TORRES and GEORG 1956, FLÓRIÁN and FARKAS 1958, ALTERAS and CONU 1962, DVOŘÁK and OTČENÁŠEK, 1964, GIP 1964). Infection of cat, dog, mouse and man are probably of bird origin. Recently, isolation of this fungus has been reported by American authors from Puerto Rico (TORRES and GEORG 1956). LONDERO, FISCHMAN and RAMOS (1964), when reviewing Brazilian cases, proved that this infection occurs in three states — Minas Gerais, Guanabara and Sao Paulo. They observed their own case in Rio Grande do Sul. Its presence in Czechoslovakia has been recorded by DVOŘÁK and OTČENÁŠEK (1962), in Hungary by FLÓRIÁN and FARKAS (1958), in Rumania by ALTERAS and CONU (1962), in Yugoslavia by ČUTURIĆ and RICHTER (1965), in Finland by PÄTIÄLÄ (1951), in Sweden by GIP (1964). In the review by COUDERT (1964), the occurrence of *T. gallinae* in France, Spain and in the U.S.S.R. is reported. This dermatophyte seems to have a more extensive geographical distribution.

Brief characteristics of the disease

The lesions are located on the featherless parts of the head, especially on the comb and the wattles, but have also been reported from the skin on the cheeks, the lid, from the submandibular region (ČUTURIĆ and RICHTER 1965) and from the pericloacal region (SPESIVTSEVA 1962). Lesions are rarely found on the base of the beak.

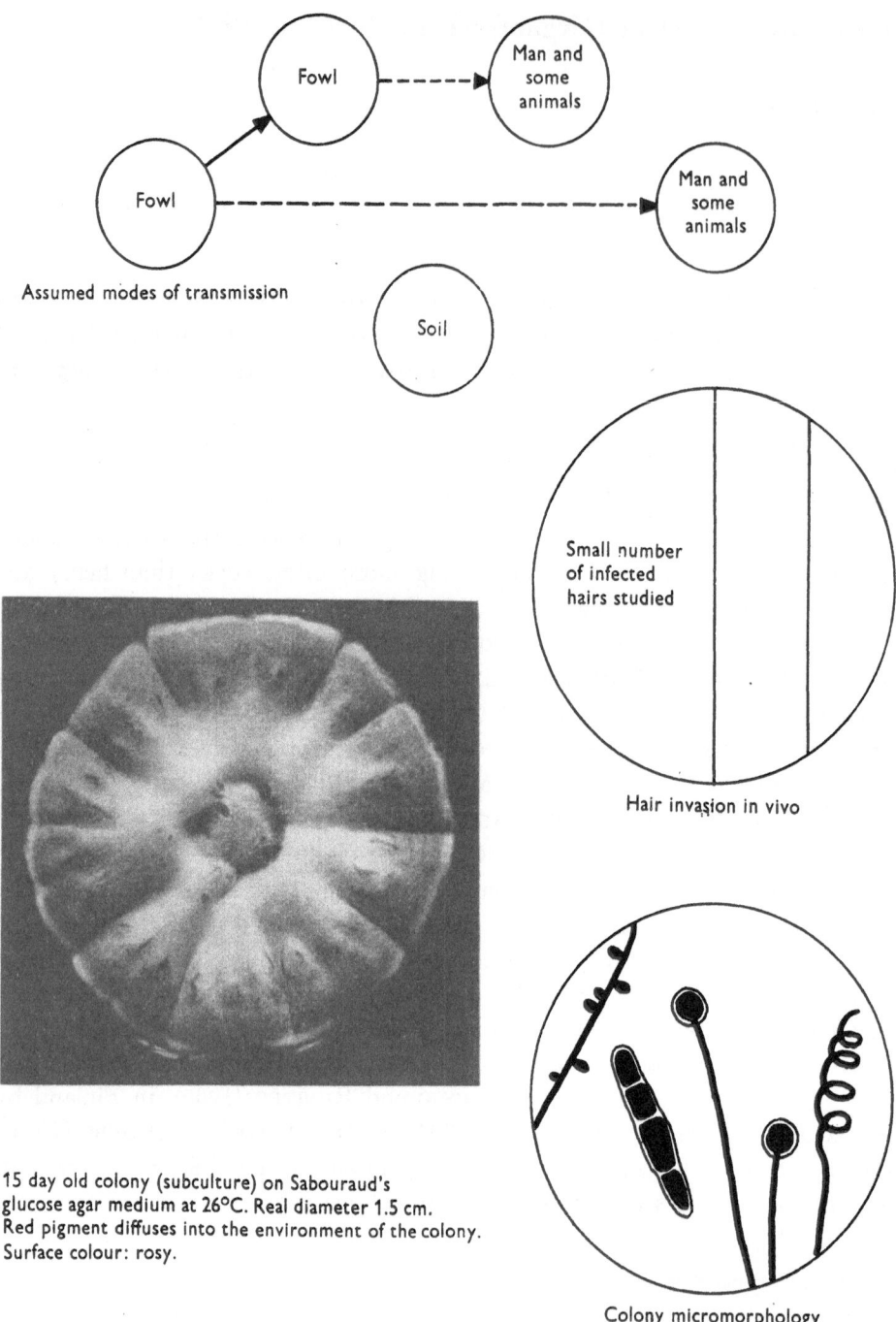

Assumed modes of transmission

Small number
of infected
hairs studied

Hair invasion in vivo

15 day old colony (subculture) on Sabouraud's
glucose agar medium at 26°C. Real diameter 1.5 cm.
Red pigment diffuses into the environment of the colony.
Surface colour: rosy.

Colony micromorphology

Fig. 20. *Trichophyton gallinae* (Mégnin) Silva et Benham 1952. World wide registered
dermatophyte, attacking mainly fowl.

These lesions form thick, white crusts on the comb and wattles. If the disease becomes generalized, the entire head is covered with minute powdered scales, sometimes even extending over the neck and body (AINSWORTH 1954). Feathers fall out from the infected parts and the chickens smell mouldy (HILBRICH 1958). Opaque crusts on the lids sometimes cause the closing of the lids (ČUTURIĆ and RICHTER 1965). When the disease spreads from the head and the neck to the other parts of the body, circular plaques are being formed and peeling occurs at their periphery. Through the heavy loss of feathers the chickens emaciate and sometimes die without other evidence of pathological changes (EL-FIKI 1959).

The crusts forming a continuous yellowish layer on the combs deeply penetrate the skin and the subcutaneous tissues; this may even cause a deep necrosis resulting in the loss of some parts of the comb. Sometimes, sloughing causes deep furrows and pits in the comb, which becomes deformed and swollen at the edges. Some authors (SPESIVTSEVA 1964) differentiate between the scutellate and the generalized form of this disease. If the lesions spread over a wider area, the chickens become unable to utilize their food and, under these conditions, lose weight, develop anemia and eventually die.

In man, tinea capitis, tinea corporis, exceptionally tinea cruris and tinea unguium have been observed.

Direct microscopy

In skin scales, branched, septate hyphae somewhere shortly coiled or twisted and arthrospores in grape-like clusters or chains are present. The arthrospores may be circular, measuring $6-8$ μm diameter. Round the feathers formations resembling favic scutula containing mycelium and arthrospores may be present. Hair invasion of the endoectothrix type with small or large extrapillar spores.

Colony macromorphology

The colony attains a diameter of $10-25$ mm at the end of 10 days. AJELLO (1963) reports rapid growth; probably some strains grow rapidly. The mature colony (after 15 days) may have a regularly circular to asteroid ground plan. Sometimes, irregularly asteroid or polygonal colonies develop. The surface may be velvety to hairy (woolly, fluffy), flat or raised, more or less wrinkled and folded. The centre may be umbilicated or depressed. In older colonies cracks can appear. The surface is white to grey, rosy, red (especially in older cultures), the reverse side is rosy, carmine, dark blood red, sometimes terracotta. Subculture can be free of pigment. The typical sign is the production of diffusible strawberry-red pigment.

Colony micromorphology

The slender branched, septate hyphae may be almost sterile. Some strains produce ovoid, clavate to pyriform microconidia (1—2 by 2—4 μm), scattered along the sides of the simple hyphae (acladium type). Macroconidia can be absent or produced in limited numbers. Sometimes, they are abundant. They are clavate, cylindro-clavate to cigar-shaped, smooth with thin walls, 2—10 cells, measuring 6—10 by 15—56 μm. No abnormal structures were observed in our strains (chandeliers, nodular bodies, pectinate hyphae, racquets or spirals). Only chlamydospores were noted (5 μm). Some strains evidently produce spirals.

Differential diagnosis

Sometimes, *T. gallinae* must be differentiated from *T. megninii* and *T. rubrum*.

Experimental pathogenicity

The cultures are always pathogenic for chickens, guinea-pigs, mice and rabbits. If combs are inoculated, lesions similar to those from a natural infection soon develop. Lesions in guinea-pigs become heavily crusted after 7 days, surrounded by areas of erythema.

Nutritional requirements

No special requirements. *T. gallinae* grows relatively well on media containing NH_4NO_3 as the sole source of nitrogen. Spore production is stimulated by adding thiamine and yeast extract to the medium.

Zoophilic dermatophytes commonly attacking man

With the exception of *M. canis*, which we have never isolated, all other dermatophytes listed here have been commonly isolated by us from various animals and man. These dermatophytes are relatively very common in our country.

Microsporon canis Bodin, 1902

Perfect state: *Veronaia felinea* Benedek, 1961*.

Synonyms: *Microsporum felineum* Mewborn, 1902; *Microsporon equinum* Sabouraud, 1907; *Microsporum caninum* (Bodin) Sabouraud, 1908; *Sabouraudites lanosus* Ota et Langeron, 1923; *Microsporum Stillianus* Benedek, 1937; *Microsporum auranticum* Conant, 1937; *Microsporum pseudolanosum* Conant, 1937; *Microsporum simiae* Conant, 1937; *Microsporum obesum* Conant, 1937.

Distribution

Saprophytic habitat and source of infection unknown. DVOŘÁK and OTČENÁŠEK (1964) record a list of those hosts of this dermatophyte, identified up to the present: cat, cattle, chinchilla, dog, donkey, guinea-pig, horse, lion, man, monkey, rabbit, sheep, swine. Recently, infection in the goat has been recorded (AUSTWICK 1966). It seems to cause very frequently and perhaps mainly dermatophytoses in the cat. Severe skin lesions may be produced in the kitten; in mature cats, fluorescent hairs are sometimes the only sign of infection so that they are true carriers of this fungus infection (KRAL 1960). The second most frequently attacked animal is the dog. Infection of other animals seems to be uncommon (GEORG 1960, BÜHLMAN and RIETH 1962, GEORG 1964). Human cases are relatively frequent and are mostly of animal origin. They are very often observed in children. The reason for this is not only their higher

---

*   Single report by BENEDEK (1961).

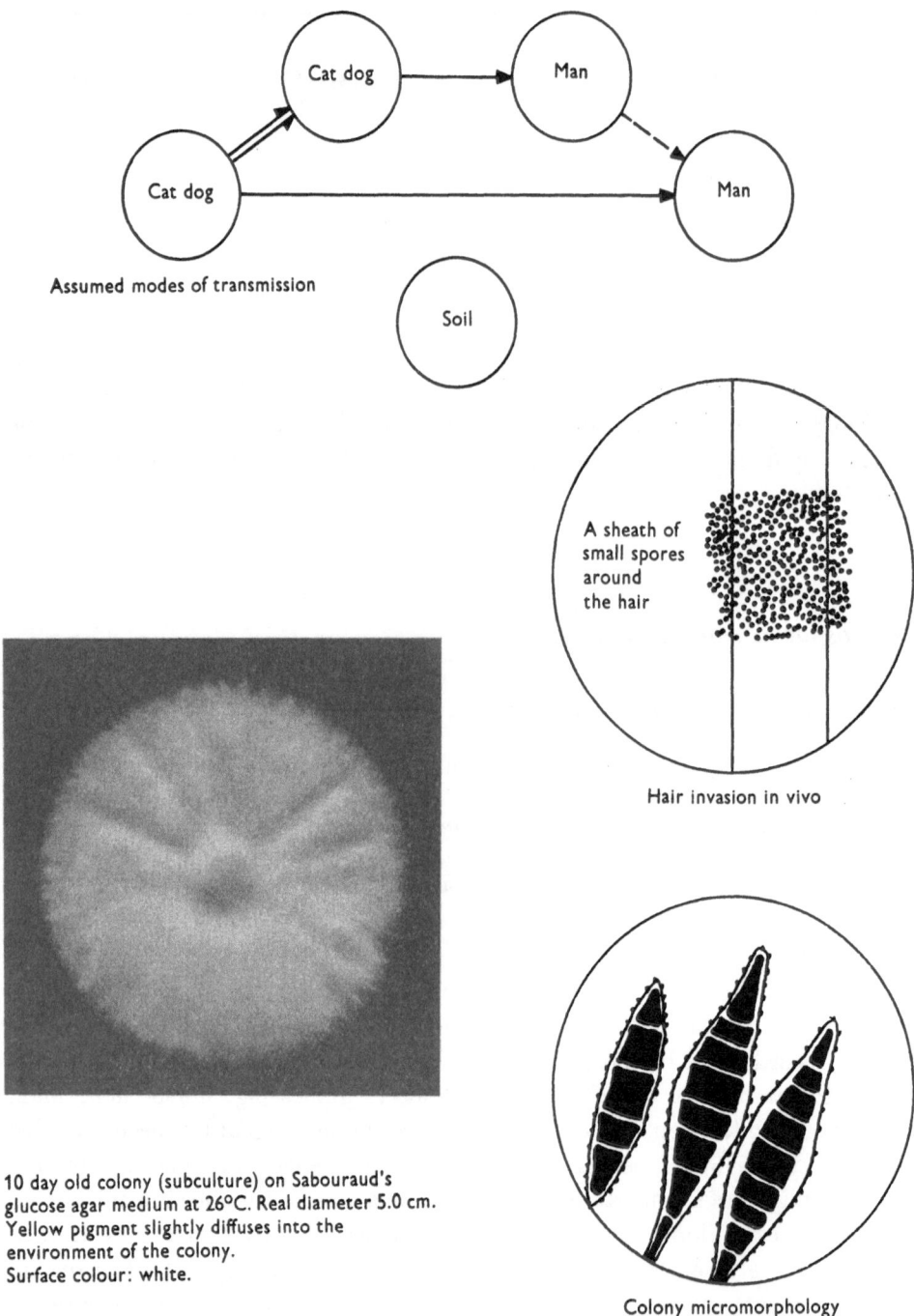

Assumed modes of transmission

A sheath of
small spores
around
the hair

Hair invasion in vivo

10 day old colony (subculture) on Sabouraud's
glucose agar medium at 26°C. Real diameter 5.0 cm.
Yellow pigment slightly diffuses into the
environment of the colony.
Surface colour: white.

Colony micromorphology

Fig. 21. *Microsporon canis* Bodin 1902. World wide registered dermatophyte, attacking frequently cat, dog and man.

susceptibility, but also the closer contact of children with cats and dogs. Man to man transmission is possible but rare (GEORG 1964). The cat seems to be the commonest source of infection. *M. canis* is most contagious among cats and may be responsible for almost a 100% of the superficial infection of cats in urban areas (CONROY 1964). AJELLO (1962) placed *M. canis* among the cosmopolitan species. This has also been confirmed by recent reports. In Czechoslovakia, *M. canis* is clearly not endemic while, on the contrary, in some countries it is very common.

Brief characteristics of the disease

Hairs, skin and claws may be affected. Young animals seem to be more susceptible to infection, but this disease has also been recorded from animals older than 5 years.

In the dog, pathological changes occur on the head, the trunk, the extremities; occasionally also the tail and claws may be affected.

At first, hairs are shed from the lesion, which then becomes covered with scales and crusts. The skin under the pealed off crust is erythematous. Often, the foci are large, of irregular shape and inflamed. The unpigmented skin is bright red especially at the periphery. A mild pruritus may occur (KRAL 1964). Sometimes, there is very little inflammatory reaction, the lesion is characterized by thickened skin and brittle hairs, which can easily be pulled out (SPESIVTSEVA 1964).

JAKSCH (1963) gave a general description of two forms of this disease. The first occurs in young, less than a year old dogs and is characterized by mild inflammatory patches on the skin, which is hardly distinguishable from the healthy skin. Hairs pull out easily and circular foci of 10—20 mm occur on the bold places. The surface of the skin becomes covered with light, minute scales. The second form found on dogs older than one year is characterized by oval to circular foci of 15—30 mm, raised above the surface of the skin. Sometimes, these foci are covered with silvery, smooth scales, sometimes they are covered with pus.

In cats, the disease is located on similar sites as in the dog. On the head it is found most frequently on the ear lobes, round the eyes and on the lips.

The lesions are circular and characterized by loss of hair and the formation of greyish-white scales. The unpigmented skin is reddish (KRAL 1964). CONROY (1964) described the following clinical forms:

1. Bright, light green fluorescence (Wood-light) with no visible lesion;

2. Hyperpigmented, flat or slightly raised patch with local alopecia and stubble hairs;

3. Lesion covered by a heavy grey crust with stubble hairs and oozing erythematous base;
4. Generalized distribution of small serosanguineous crusts without alopecia;
5. Onychomycosis (infection of the claws).

In children, the lesions are situated on the exposed areas of the skin, frequently on the scalp. Infection of adults is occasional and usually localised on face and neck. However, tinea barbae, pedis and unguium have also been reported.

Direct microscopy

The hair invasion is of the endoectothrix type with small (2—3 to 5 µm) extrapillar spores. In skin scales, branched septate hyphae more or less arthrosporulated are found.

Colony macromorphology

The colony attains a diameter of 35—55 mm at the end of 10 days. The mature colony (after 10 days) has mostly a regularly circular to asteroid ground plan. The surface is at first silky, later dense. It can be hairy, fluffy, cottony, woolly, velvety powdered. There is no great tendency to wrinkle. Sometimes, several radial furrows develop. The colour of the colony changes with age. The aerial part of the colony is at first white, salmon, pale lemon yellow to lemon yellow or bright brownish yellow. The reverse side is mostly saffron yellow, lemon yellow to yellow, later dull orange brown. The soluble pigment diffuses sometimes markedly into the periphery of the colony. It is pale lemon yellow to lemon yellow. Only some strains are unpigmented.

Colony micromorphology

The most important diagnostic feature is the presence of abundant spindle-shaped macroconidia with pointed tapering ends, rough, thick walls, 5—15 cells, measuring 6—20 by 30—150 µm. In primocultures microconidia (ovoid, clavate to pyriform, 2—3 by 3·5 µm) are occasionally present in limited numbers. They are sessile-borne, en thyrses (acladium type). Racquets are almost always produced. Nodular bodies, spirals or pectinate hyphae and chlamydospores are scarce, if present. Chlamydospores may be produced in remarkable numbers in older cultures.

Experimental pathogenicity

The cultures are pathogenic for a wide scale of animals. Infection of guinea-pigs results in heavily crusted lesions after 15—20 days, which heal spontaneously within 5 weeks.

Keratinolysis of hairs in vitro

M. canis lyses the hairs of man rectangularly to its long axis, the hairs of goat, guinea-pig and mouse coaxially and the hairs of cattle, dog and horse both rectangularly and coaxially.

Nutritional requirements

The fungus grows well on rice grains.

Atypical strains

Recently, KLOKKE and DE VRIES (1963) and KABEN (1964) isolated from monkeys atypical strains resembling *M. obesum* Conant, 1937, which have been more recently considered to be a synonym of *M. canis*. KABEN (1964), giving the characteristics of these strains and of the strains by SEELIGER, BISPING and BRANDT (1963), also isolated from the monkey, identified it as *M. audouinii*. It has been concluded that the first two strains are closely related to *M. obesum*. Macroscopically these strains are similar to the typical *M. canis*, however, the measurements of the macroconidia have shown some constant differences.

Trichophyton mentagrophytes (**Robin**) **Blanchard, 1896**

Perfect state: not known.

Synonyms: *Microsporum mentagrophytes* Robin, 1853; *Trichophyton gypseum* Bodin, 1902; *Trichophyton granulosum* Sabouraud, 1909; *Trichophyton radians* Sabouraud, 1909; *Trichophyton asteroides* Sabouraud, 1910.

Many of the synonyms were given to varieties (e.g. *T. mentagrophytes* var. *asteroides*, var. *granulosum*). Some authors placed here also *T. equinum*, *T. interdigitale* and *T. quinckeanum* (e.g. CONANT et al. 1954). At the International Congress of Dermatology in Stockholm (1957) GEORG submitted a system which includes *T. equinum* as a valid species. The arrangement of *T. interdigitale* and *T. quinckeanum* to *T. mentagrophytes* has not been commonly accepted (e.g. GÖTZ 1964, NOVÁK and GALGÓCZY 1963, DONALD and BROWN 1964). It is most probable that before *T. terrestre* has been described, some of its properties had been ascribed to *T. mentagrophytes*.

Varieties: *T. mentagrophytes* var. *erinacei*; *T. mentagrophytes* var. *interdigitale*; *T. mentagrophytes* var. *quinckeanum*.

Distribution

Saprophytic habitat and source of infection is not known, although the soil may be suspected (EVOLCEANU, ALTERAS and COJOCARU 1964). DVOŘÁK and OTČENÁŠEK (1964) record a list of those hosts of this dermatophyte identified up to the present: cat, cattle, chinchilla, dog, donkey, fox, goat, guinea-pig, hedgehog, horse, kangaroo, man, monkey, mouse, mule, muskrat, opossum, polecat, rabbit, rat, sheep, squirrel, swine, chicken. REFAI (1966) reported the infection of buffalo, MAKMIKYA (1963) of nutria, MARAIS and OLIVIER (1965) of porcupine. This shows the very wide spectrum of hosts known up to the present. There is not sufficient evidence yet, which of the animals is the most frequent host and important source of infection. *T. mentagrophytes* has repeatedly been isolated from hairs of apparently healthy animals, e.g. dog, hedgehog, mouse (TAYLOR, RADCLIFFE and VAN PEENEN 1964, CONNOLE 1963, ENGLISH 1964 a.o.) but, in some cases, the correctness of the identification seemed doubtful. It is possible that small mammals are the true source of infection of animals and man (GEORG 1960, 1964). *T. mentagrophytes* seems to belong to the dermatophytes which are not too important for veterinary medicine. Perhaps only horses and donkeys are relatively frequently attacked (KRAL 1960). In eastern Bohemia (1962 to 1964) it has been found as the rare cause of cattle and guinea-pig ringworm (DVOŘÁK, OTČENÁŠEK and KOMÁREK 1965). It is an important cause of human dermatophytoses in our country (DVOŘÁK and OTČENÁŠEK 1965). In some countries throughout the world, human cases are very common especially in rural areas (AJELLO 1962). In eastern Bohemia (1952—1953), *T. mentagrophytes* has been frequently isolated (21%) after the clinical examination of patients suffering from dermatophytosis. After *T. rubrum*, this was the second most important dermatophyte attacking man. In 1962—1963, *T. mentagrophytes* became third in importance after *T. rubrum* and *T. verrucosum* (9% of people suffering from dermatophytoses) (DVOŘÁK and OTČENÁŠEK 1965).

Brief characteristics of the disease

In cattle, the lesions are located on the head, neck and trunk, preferably on the anterior part of the body. They are characterized by minute, mostly circular foci with loss of hair. The surface of the lesions is covered with small scales resembling bran. Crusty lesions, so typical for dermatophytoses caused by *T. verrucosum*, are mostly absent.

In horses, the lesions are not only found on the head, neck and trunk, but also on the extremities and close to the base of the tail. They are mostly circular or irregularly circular in shape, covered with thick grey crusts and debris of hair. At an early stage, papules, vesicles and pustules may occur. These break open at a later stage and crusts are formed from their contents.

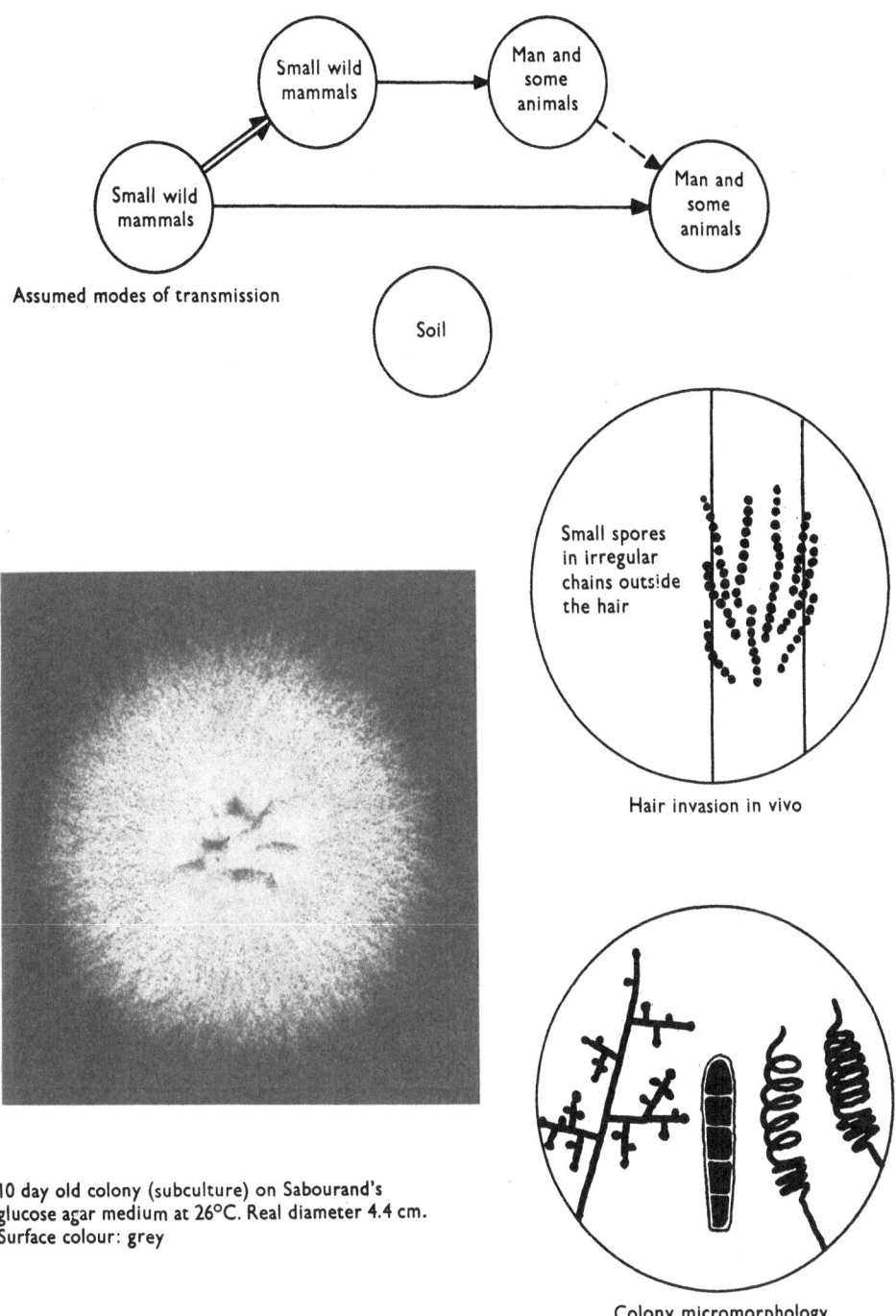

Assumed modes of transmission

Soil

Small spores
in irregular
chains outside
the hair

Hair invasion in vivo

10 day old colony (subculture) on Sabourand's
glucose agar medium at 26°C. Real diameter 4.4 cm.
Surface colour: grey

Colony micromorphology

Fig. 22. *Trichophyton mentagrophytes* (Robin) Blanchard 1896. World wide registered dermatophyte, attacking frequently small wild mammals, various other animals
and man.

These changes may be accompanied by pruritus (KRAL and SCHWARTZMANN 1964).

In dogs, circular, scaly foci with thickened erythematous rims occur. Here again, the initial stage is characterized by pustular and vesicular efflorescences, which are drying up into crusts. Lesions, covered with these crusts may simulate demodicosis (KRAL and SCHWARTZMANN 1964).

In pigs, the foci are covered with brown crusts. The reverse side of these lesions is reddish (GINTHER et al. 1964).

In rabbits, the most frequently affected parts of the head are the ear lobes, the nose and the eyes. The lesions are mostly covered with crusts or alopecia develops, covered with epidermal scales.

In fur-bearing animals, superficial or deep inflammatory reactions occur. The superficial forms are characterized by alopecia foci with scales. The deep forms are accompanied by the formation of a purulent exudate.

The lesions in man may be located elsewhere on the body surface (tinea capitis, barbae, corporis, manus, perigenitalis, pedis and unguium). In children, they seem to occur most frequently as tinea capitis, in adults as tinea barbae and corporis (forearms). Tinea manum, pedis, cruris and unguium may be found occasionally. No fluorescence of infected hairs.

Direct microscopy

The hair invasion is of the endoectothrix type with small extrapillar spores (3—5 µm). In skin scales, branched, septate hyphae more or less arthrosporulated are found.

Colony macromorphology

The colony attains a diameter of 25—45 mm after 10 days. The mature colony (after 10 days) has mostly a regularly circular to asteroid ground plan. The surface is heavily granular, sometimes velvety powdered. There is little tendency to wrinkle. Mostly, the colony is entirely flat-granulomatous, directly covering the medium. Sometimes, a depression with or without irregular folds occurs in its centre. Some colonies develop a central umbilicus. Radial furrows are formed only exceptionally. The aerial part of the colony can be white to grey, pale rosy, salmon, apricot, pale lemon yellow, violet or lilac, specially in the centre. The reverse side is mostly terracotta, sienna or pale lemon yellow.

Colony micromorphology

All strains produce numerous spherical to ovoid microconidia (2—2·5 by 2—4·5 µm), mostly in compound sporiferous hyphae, en grappes. Sometimes, macroconidia are not found, but in some strains they are present in relatively high numbers. They are clavate to cigar-shaped, smooth, with thin walls, 3—8 cells, measuring 5—12 by 12—55 μm. Spirals can be either abundant or rare. Nodular bodies, racquets, pectinate hyphae and chlamydospores are found.

Differential diagnosis

Sometimes *T. mentagrophytes* must be differentiated from *T. equinum* or *T. simii*.

Experimental pathogenicity

The cultures are pathogenic for a wide scale of laboratory animals. Infection of guinea-pigs results, after 10 days, in erythematous and crusted lesions, which spontaneously heal in 5 weeks.

Keratinolysis of hairs in vitro

T. mentagrophytes attacks the hairs of dog and man rectangularly to its axis. Coaxial keratinolysis occurs in the hairs of cattle, goat, guinea-pig and mouse.

Nutritional requirements

No special requirements. It does not require thiamine and inositol.

Atypical strains

GEORG and MAECHLING (1949) reported *T. mentagrophytes* var. *nodular*, a mutant with brilliant orange-red pigment isolated in nine cases of ringworm of the skin and nails. The aerial mycelium is fluffy and submerged mycelium is filled with numerous nodular bodies.

Trichophyton mentagrophytes (Robin) Blanchard var. *erinacei* Smith et Marples, 1963

Isolations have been reported from hedgehogs and infected human contacts in New Zealand and Great Britain by MARPLES and SMITH (1960), LA TOUCHE and FORSTER (1963), SMITH and MARPLES (1963), ENGLISH (1964), ENGLISH, SMITH and RUSH-MUNRO (1964), QUAIFE (1966). The colony grows with similar rapidity as *T. mentagrophytes*. The mature colony (after 10 days) is circular, finely powdered and flat. The surface is white to creamy, the reverse side brilliant lemon yellow. Microconidia are elongated, 1·2 by 4·9 μm. Macroconidia irregular in shape and size, smooth, with thin walls, 2—6 cells. Spirals absent. Cultures pathogenic for guinea-pigs.

Trichophyton mentagrophytes (Robin) Blanchard var. interdigitale Priestley, 1917

Some authors consider it to be a valid species. Known also as *T. Kaufmann-Wolfii* Ota, 1922.

Distribution

Findings in animal lesions and its pathogenic role (CETIN, TAHSINOGLU and VOLKAN 1965) must be confirmed. Saprophytic habitat and source of infection unknown. Probably mainly interhuman propagation. Human infection very common, occurring throughout the world. Sometimes found in interdigital spaces of human feet without apparent pathological changes. Tinea corporis, tinea manus, cruris and unguium have also been observed, tinea capitis and barbae are extremely rare. It does not attack hairs.

Colony macromorphology

The colony attains 20—40 mm in diameter at the end of 10 days. The mature colony (after 10 days) has mostly a regular, circular ground plan. It is velvety to fluffy, mostly without furrows. The surface colour can be white, grey, salmon or pale lemon yellow. The reverse side can be unpigmented, saffron yellow, terra-cotta or rusty.

Colony micromorphology

Micromorphology can be poor. Macroconidia are not produced. Microconidia are found, but normally in limited numbers. They are ovoid, clavate to pyriform, 2 by 2·5 μm. Spirals can be abundant. Especially in older cultures, chlamydospores have been observed.

Differential diagnosis

T. mentagrophytes var. *interdigitale* must sometimes be differentiated from *T. rubrum*.

Experimental pathogenecity

Normally, typical strains are apathogenic.

Keratinolysis of hairs in vitro

T. mentagrophytes var. *interdigitale* does not differ in this sense from *T. mentagrophytes*.

Trichophyton mentagrophytes (Robin) Blanchard
var. *quinckeanum* (Quincke 1885) Blanchard 1896

Synonyms: *Achorion quinckeanum* Quincke, 1885; *Sabouraudites quinckeanus* Ota et Langeron, 1923; *Microsporum quinckeanum* Guiart et Grigorakis, 1928; *Achorion muris* Dodge, 1935; *T. gypseum* Bodin var. *quinckeanum* Blanchard, 1896.

The precise study by LA TOUCHE (1960) confirms this conception. However, its inclusion as a synonym or variety of *T. mentagrophytes* has not been commonly accepted and some prominent mycologists such as GÖTZ (1964) consider it to be a valid species. Studies by BROWN and DONALD (1964), DONALD and BROWN (1964) have shown that the existing differences warrant to give it a separate identity as a variety of *T. mentagrophytes*. In the opinion of BALABANOFF and KASAROV (1963), it is a valid species in synonymy with *T. niveum* Sabouraud, 1910.

Distribution

Saprophytic habitat and source of infection unknown, although soil may be suspected (EVOLCEANU, ALTERAS and COJOCARU 1964). DVOŘÁK and OTČENÁŠEK (1964) record a list of those hosts of this dermatophyte, identified up to the present: cat, cattle, dog, fox, horse, man, mouse, rabbit, rat and sheep. We have isolated a typical strain from a dermatophytic lesion of a hen (DVOŘÁK, OTČENÁŠEK and KOMÁREK 1965). The most important host, frequently the source of infection for other animals, seems to be the mouse. In fact other animals are not very frequently attacked. By contrast, lesions due to this dermatophyte are relatively often reported in man (e.g. KABEN and PLÖTZ 1962, RDZANEK, WEYMAN-RZUCIDLO and POHORECKA 1963, ALTERAS 1965). In the last decade it has been found in Europe (e.g. England, France, Germany, Poland and Rumania), in Canada and Australia. We have isolated it several times from dermatophytic lesions of cattle, chicken and man in eastern Bohemia. It seems that this dermatophyte is distributed especially in rural areas throughout the world.

Brief characteristics of the disease

T. mentagrophytes var. *quinckeanum* causes a typical ringworm in the mouse, commonly referred to as "mouse favus". Favic scutula are often found in rodents. In other animals and man, the lesions may be similar to those observed in other dermatophytoses. In man, tinea capitis, barbae and corporis are reported. Also tinea cruris and unguium have been observed occasionally.

Direct microscopy

Hair invasion of the endoectothrix type with small extrapillar spores (2—5 μm). Sometimes, endothrix hair invasion has been observed.

Colony macromorphology

The colony attains a diameter of 10—30 mm at the end of 10 days. The mature colony (after 10 days) has a regularly or irregularly asteroid or polygonal ground plan. The surface is velvety to velvety powdered. The colonies of most strains are more or less wrinkled. The aerial part of the colony is white to grey, pale rosy, pale lemon yellow, lilac to purplish. The reverse is carmine, dark blood red to rusty. The soluble pigment produces a ring round the colony. Sometimes, pigmentation occurs in patches.

Colony micromorphology

All strains produce numerous spherical, predominantly ovoid, clavate to pyriform microconidia (2—4 by 2—7 μm). Macroconidia are not always found, but when present in some strains, they are clavate to spindle-shaped, smooth, with thin walls, 2—11 cells and measure 4—11 by 18—76 μm. The terminal cells are often pointed. Filiform appendages from the terminal cell are regularly present. Spirals may be either abundant or rare. Sometimes, nodular bodies have been found; chlamydospores of about 15 μm have been frequently observed.

Experimental pathogenicity

The cultures are pathogenic for a wide scale of especially young laboratory animals (guinea-pig, mouse, rabbit). Infection of guinea-pig results in erythematous and crusted lesions after 10 days. In the mouse, a typical scutula can develop. The hairs can fluoresce in yellowish – green colour in Wood's light.

Comparison of *T. mentagrophytes* and its varieties

Growth	*Trichophyton mentagrophytes*	*T. ment.* var. *erinacei*	*T. ment.* var. *interdigitale*	*T. ment.* var. *quinckeanum*
on soil and keratin				
at pH 4·0	+++	+	++	?
at 35°C	++	±	++	?
Hair invasion	+	++	+	?
Spirals	+	+	0	+
Pigment	+++	0	+	++/0
	red to brown	brilliant lemon yellow	yellow brown to rose	carmine dark blood red to rusty

Trichophyton verrucosum Bodin, 1902

Perfect state: not known.

Synonyms: *T. album* Sabouraud, 1908; *T. ochraceum* Sabouraud, 1910; *T. discoides* Sabouraud, 1910.

AINSWORTH and GEORG (1954) recommended the following nomenclature:

T. verrucosum Bodin var. *verrucosum* (Sabouraud) Georg,
T. verrucosum Bodin var. *album* (Sabouraud) Georg,
T. verrucosum Bodin var. *ochraceum* (Sabouraud) Georg.

Some authors considered it to be identical with *T. schoenleinii* (e. g. CONANT et al. 1954). At the International Congress of Dermatology in Stockholm (1957) Georg submitted a system which includes *T. verrucosum* as a valid species.

Distribution

Saprophytic habitat and source of infection unknown. Occasional finding in the soil is no proof of its saprophytic origin. DVOŘÁK and OTČENÁŠEK (1964) record a list of those hosts of this dermatophyte identified up to the present: canary, chicken, cat, cattle, dog, donkey, dromedary, goat, horse, mule, sheep, swine. Primary attacks have mainly been recorded from cattle, infection of other animals is uncommon and occurs only in connection with infected cattle. Human cases are relatively frequent among children and adults especially in rural areas. Ringworm of cattle and man caused by this fungus is world wide distributed and very frequent in some countries. In eastern Bohemia (1962—1964) it was found as the common cause of cattle ringworm. It has also been isolated from ringworm-like lesions from chickens, dogs, horses and one pig (OTČENÁŠEK, DVOŘÁK and KOMÁREK 1964, DVOŘÁK, OTČENÁŠEK and KOMÁREK 1965). It is also considered to be a very important agent of human dermatophytoses in Czechoslovakia. Recently, there has been a marked increase in its frequency of occurrence and, at the present, it is after *T. rubrum* the most frequent cause of human ringworm (DVOŘÁK and OTČENÁŠEK 1965).

Brief characteristics of the disease

In cattle, the lesions are mostly distributed over the whole body, prefering the head, the neck, the sides and the back. In calves, most of the lesions are found on the head, sometimes forming a brim round the eyes, covering the cheeks and the forehead and also occurring on both sides of the ear lobes. In some instances, lesions have been found on the extremities and the tail. In adult cattle, circular small foci are distributed over the whole surface of the

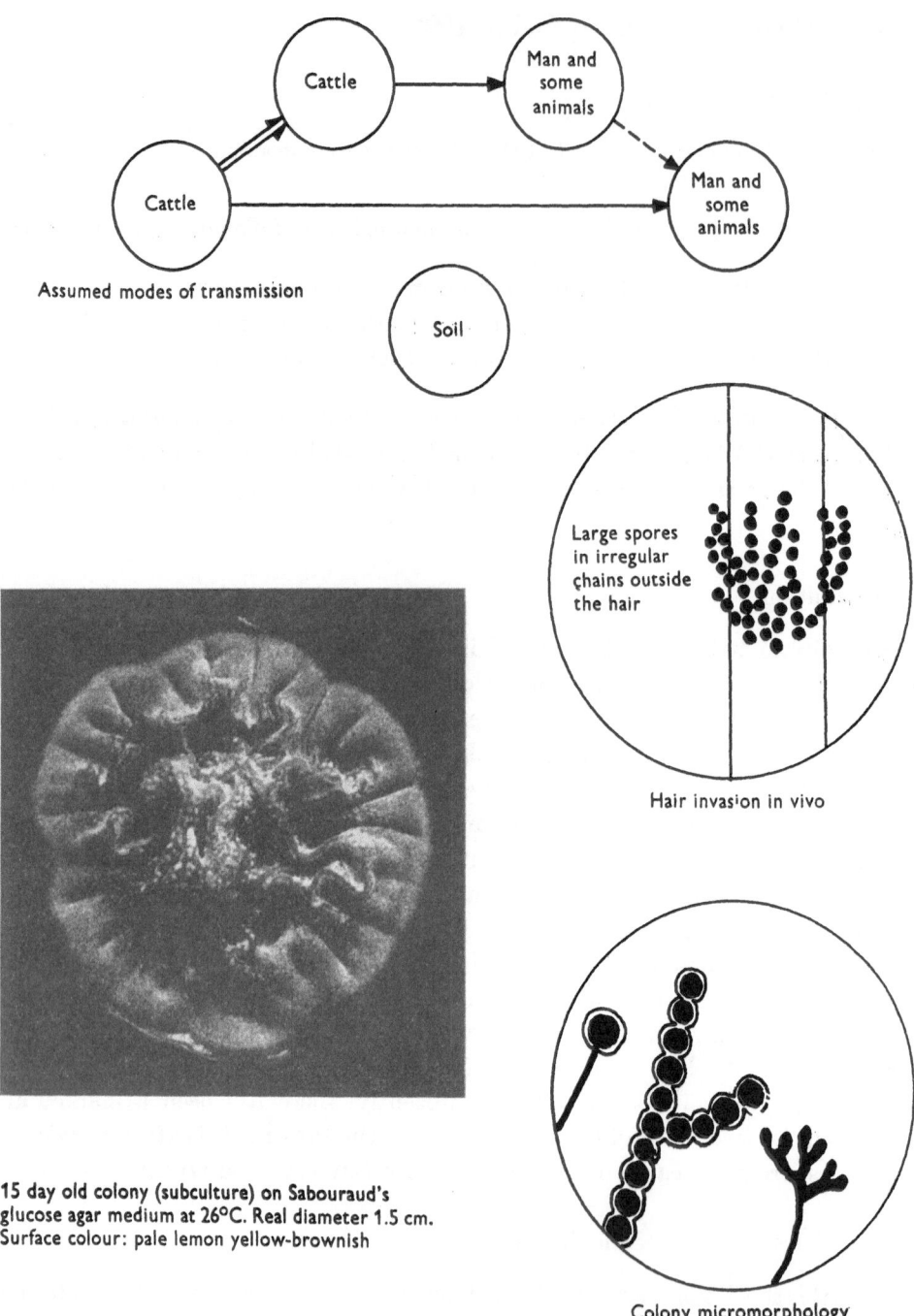

Assumed modes of transmission

Large spores
in irregular
chains outside
the hair

Hair invasion in vivo

15 day old colony (subculture) on Sabouraud's
glucose agar medium at 26°C. Real diameter 1.5 cm.
Surface colour: pale lemon yellow-brownish

Colony micromorphology

Fig. 23. *Trichophyton verrucosum* Bodin 1902. World wide registered dermatophyte,
attacking mainly cattle and man.

body which, at first, are not very marked and typical. The hairs fall out from the infected places or are stuck together in tufts by the discharge of the inflamed skin. After desiccation of the exudate, crusts are formed, which spread in irregular patterns into the environment. The foci vary in size, being of circular or irregular shape. Sometimes, especially in the adult cattle, the foci are minute and circular, characterized by the loss of hair and the formation of fine scales. Some foci resemble abrasions or loss of hair after soiling. Some authors (e.g. TORDA and MOLNÁR 1962, SPECIVTSEVA 1964) distinguish a superficial and a deep form of this disease. Deep forms are mostly found in young cattle. Here, the foci are covered coherently by adhering crusts, covering the reddish to yellowish brown skin. Some animals are cachectic and gain little in weight.

In sheep and goat, the foci are mostly located round the ears, the horns, at the root of the nose, on the eyelids, on the nape and round the tail, but may also occur on the back, the neck, the chest, in suckling kids on the lips (VRTIAK et al. 1962, SPESIVTSEVA 1964, KIELSTEIN and WELLER 1965 a.o.).

The affections are crusted, sometimes bleeding, confluent. Their appearance may simulate diseases caused by scabies or ecthyma contagiosa ovis (KIELSTEIN and WELLER, 1965). SPESIVTSEVA (1964) distinguishes a superficial and deep, follicular form. Other authors (e.g. KRAL and SCHWARTZMAN 1964) consider the crusty changes in sheep to be typical for this disease, whereas the affections in the goat resemble cattle lesions.

In swine, the foci are usually located on the back, the loins, the walls of the chest and on the outer side of the thigh. Pathological changes are not characterized by crusts, but by scales and sometimes by blisters (VRTIAK et al. 1962). According to SPESIVTSEVA (1964), the bristles on the attacked places have a golden sheen and the changes are accompanied by itching.

In horses, the foci are in similar location as those of *T. equinum*, attacking the neck, the saddle region, the buttock, the chest, the root of the tail and the extremities. The majority of circular foci are characterized by the loss of hair and by a finely scaly epidermis. The skin round the foci is hyperemic.

In dogs, the lesions are mostly located on the head. Characteristic are minute pustules and broken off hairs. In the later stages, the multiple foci become covered with scales and stubble hairs. Erythema is found on the unpigmented skin (KRAL and SCHWARTZMANN 1964). Some writers (SPESIVTSEVA 1964) observed the deep follicular form.

In man, *T. verrucosum* is most often identified as the cause of tinea corporis, less frequently tinea capitis and barbae. Exceptionally reported as the cause of tinea pedis.

No fluorescence of infected hairs.

Direct microscopy

The invasion of the hairs of cattle and man is nearly always of the endoecto-thrix type with large spores (3·5—10 μm). In skin scales, branched septate hyphae, more or less arthrosporulated, are found.

Colony macromorphology

The rate of growth of the colony is slow; it attains 5—15 mm in diameter after 10 days. The mature colony (after 20 days) is mostly irregular, asteroid polygonal or lobulate, only sometimes its ground plan is regular, circular to asteroid. Very often a large zone of irregular, submerged mycelium develops. The aerial part of the colony can remain underdeveloped for a long time, sometimes it is almost invisible. The colonies of some strains are membranous, more or less powdered or velvety. They may be flat or raised with a marked tendency to wrinkle. The surface colour can be grey, salmon, apricot or pale lemon yellow. The reverse can be unpigmented or salmon.

Colony micromorphology

The micromorphology is poor. The most frequent elements found are chlamy-dospores, often arranged in more or less long chains. The macroconidia are normally absent, only some strains produce them in limited numbers. They are irregular, smooth, with thin walls, 4—7 cells, measuring 4—8 by 16—50 μm. The microconidia are mostly absent, only sometimes they are found in limited numbers. They are ovoid, clavate to pyriform, 2—3 by 3—4 μm. Favic chande-liers are often present, pectinate hyphae only occasionally observed.

Differential diagnosis

T. verrucosum must sometimes be differentiated from *T. concentricum, T. schoen-leinii* and *T. yaoundei*.

Experimental pathogenicity

Pathogenic for guinea-pigs. Endoectothrix hair invasion with large spores.

Keratinolysis of hairs in vitro

T. verrucosum attacks coaxially the hairs of cattle, dog, goat, horse, mouse and man.

Nutritional requirement

Most strains require thiamine and inositol, some thiamine only.

Anthropophilic dermatophytes occasionally attacking animals

In eastern Bohemia and probably also anywhere else in Czechoslovakia we isolated hundreds of strains, which are kept in our collection. However, only in two cases a *T. rubrum*-like dermatophyte has been obtained from lesions of chimpanzees, although thousands of domestic, laboratory or wild animals have been examined. No other dermatophyte of this group have been isolated by us from animals. We identified *T. schoenleinii* only once as the causative agent of a human dermatophytosis. Only epidemics in schools due to *M. audouinii* have been studied. *T. megninii*, *T. tonsurans* and *T. violaceum* seem to have disappeared more or less rapidly from our country. With the exception of *T. tonsurans*, numerous strains of these dermatophytes are preserved in our collection without marked morphological changes.

Epidermophyton floccosum (Harz) Langeron et Milochevitch, 1930

Perfect state: not known.

Synonyms: *Trichothecium floccosum* Harz, 1870; *Epidermophyton cruris* Castellani et Chalmers, 1910; *Epidermophyton inguinale* Sabouraud, 1910.

Distribution

Saprophytic habitat and source of infection unknown. Mainly interhuman propagation probable. This species seems to be adapted for parasitic life especially in the intertriginous areas of the human body. Known also as inhabitant of the interdigital spaces of human feet without visible pathogenic changes. It causes especially tinea cruris and pedis; tinea corporis, manus and unguium have also been reported (tinea capitis is extremely rare). Until now, only one animal dermatophytosis due to this species has been recorded in the mouse (KREMPL, LAMPRECHT, and BOSSE 1964). Hairs are never invaded.

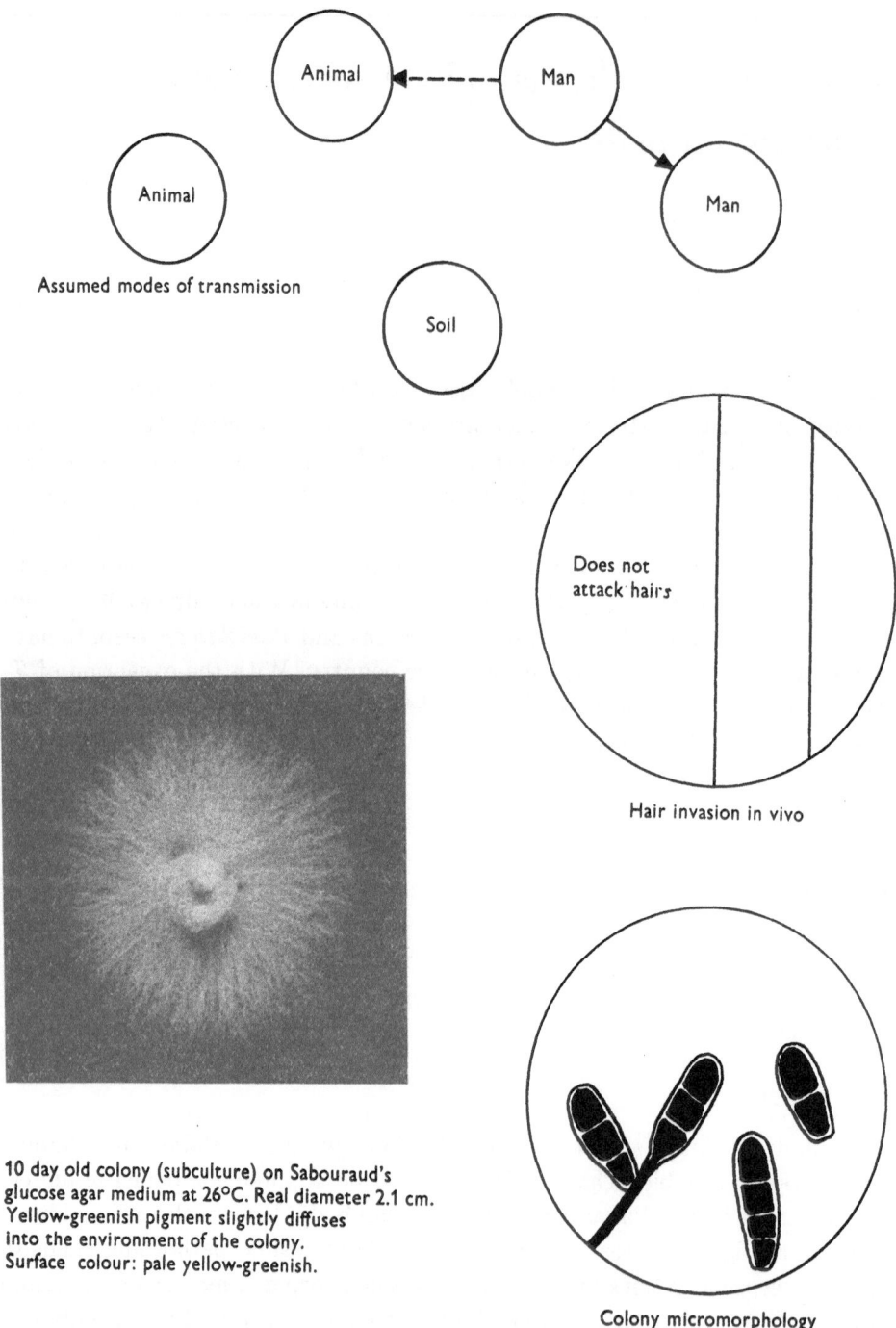

Assumed modes of transmission

Does not
attack hairs

Hair invasion in vivo

10 day old colony (subculture) on Sabouraud's
glucose agar medium at 26°C. Real diameter 2.1 cm.
Yellow-greenish pigment slightly diffuses
into the environment of the colony.
Surface colour: pale yellow-greenish.

Colony micromorphology

Fig. 24 *Epidermophyton floccosum* (Harz) Langeron et Milochevitch 1930. World
wide registered dermatophyte commonly attacking man.

Colony macromorphology

The colony attains 10—25 mm in diameter after 10 days. The mature colony
(after 15 days) has mostly a regular ground plan, circular to asteroid. It can
be membranous and powdered, velvety, velvety powdered to granular, sometimes with early appearing tufts of relatively dense white aerial hyphae (pleomorphism). The colonies form furrows and folds. The surface colour is tan to
olive green. It can be pale lemon yellow to lemon yellow, yellow, egg-yolk
yellow, pale lemon green; the yellow pigment sometimes diffuses into the
environment. The reverse side is yellowish tan, saffron yellow, pale lemon
yellow, lemon yellow, yellow, egg-yolk yellow or honey yellow.

Colony micromorphology

The most important diagnostic feature is the presence of numerous ovoid
to clavate macroconidia, smooth, with thin walls, 2—10, but mostly 2—4 cells,
measuring 5—14 by 24—85 μm. Microconidia are not produced. Nodular bodies,
pectinate hyphae, racquets and spirals are occasionally seen. Especially
in older cultures chlamydospores can be abundant.

Experimental pathogenicity

Apathogenic for laboratory animals.

Keratinolysis of hairs in vitro

E. floccosum attacks the human hairs rectangularly, the hairs of dog and goat
coaxially, the hairs of cattle and horse both coaxially and rectangularly. Mouse
hairs are not invaded.

Microsporon audouinii Gruby, 1843

Perfect state: *Veronaia audouinii* Benedek, 1961.*

Synonyms: *Microsporum velveticum* Sabouraud, 1907; *Microsporum tardum* Sabouraud,
1909; *Sabouraudites audouinii* Ota et Langeron, 1923.

M. umbonatum Sabouraud, 1907, previously listed to *M. audouinii*, has been

---

*   Single report by BENEDEK (1961).

recently suspected to be identical with *Microsporon distortum* (FLÓRIÁN, GAL-GÓCZY, NOVÁK 1964).

Distribution

Saprophytic habitat and source of infection unknown. Probably mainly human propagation. This species seems to be well adapted for parasitic life especially in the scalp of children. Tinea corporis is less frequent, tinea barbae, pedis, cruris and unguium exceptional. DVOŘÁK and OTČENÁŠEK (1964) record in their list the animal hosts of this dermatophyte: dog, guinea-pig, monkey, rabbit. Animal dermatophytoses due to this species are uncommon or rare, probably mostly of human origin. Infection of man is of world wide distribution (AJELLO 1962), somewhere very common, somewhere absent. Recently, a decrease of this infection has been observed in Europe. The hair invasion is of the endoectothrix type with small spores (2—3 μm). Bright yellowish-green fluorescence of the infected hairs.

Colony macromorphology

The colony attains 20—35 mm in diameter after 10 days. The mature colony (after 10 days) has mostly a regular ground plan, circular to asteroid. It is velvety and flat with some radial furrows. The surface colour can be snow white, pale rosy, salmon, pale lemon yellow, pale violaceous or lilac. Older colonies are brownish. The unpigmented reverse side is salmon, orange – tan, apricot to brownish with various shades.

Colony micromorphology

The macroconidia, the shape, structure and size of which are of such important diagnostic value, are usually produced in small numbers and often absent. When produced, they are irregularly developed, spindle-shaped, smooth or rough, with thin walls, 2—10 cells, measuring 8—25 by 31—190 μm. They can be indistinguishable from those produced by *M. canis*. Strains of *M. audouinii* producing numerous macroconidia have been observed, however, their arrangement to the species *M. audouinii* cannot be accepted without doubts. Almost all strains produce only a few sessile microconidia en thyrses (acladium type). They are ovoid, clavate to pyriform, measuring 1·5—3 by 2—5 μm. Nodular bodies are mostly absent, sometimes observed in limited numbers. Pectinate hyphae are few. Racquets are numerous. Some strains produce rudimentary spirals. Chlamydospores abundant especially in older cultures.

Differential diagnosis

M. audouinii must sometimes be differentiated from *M. distortum*.

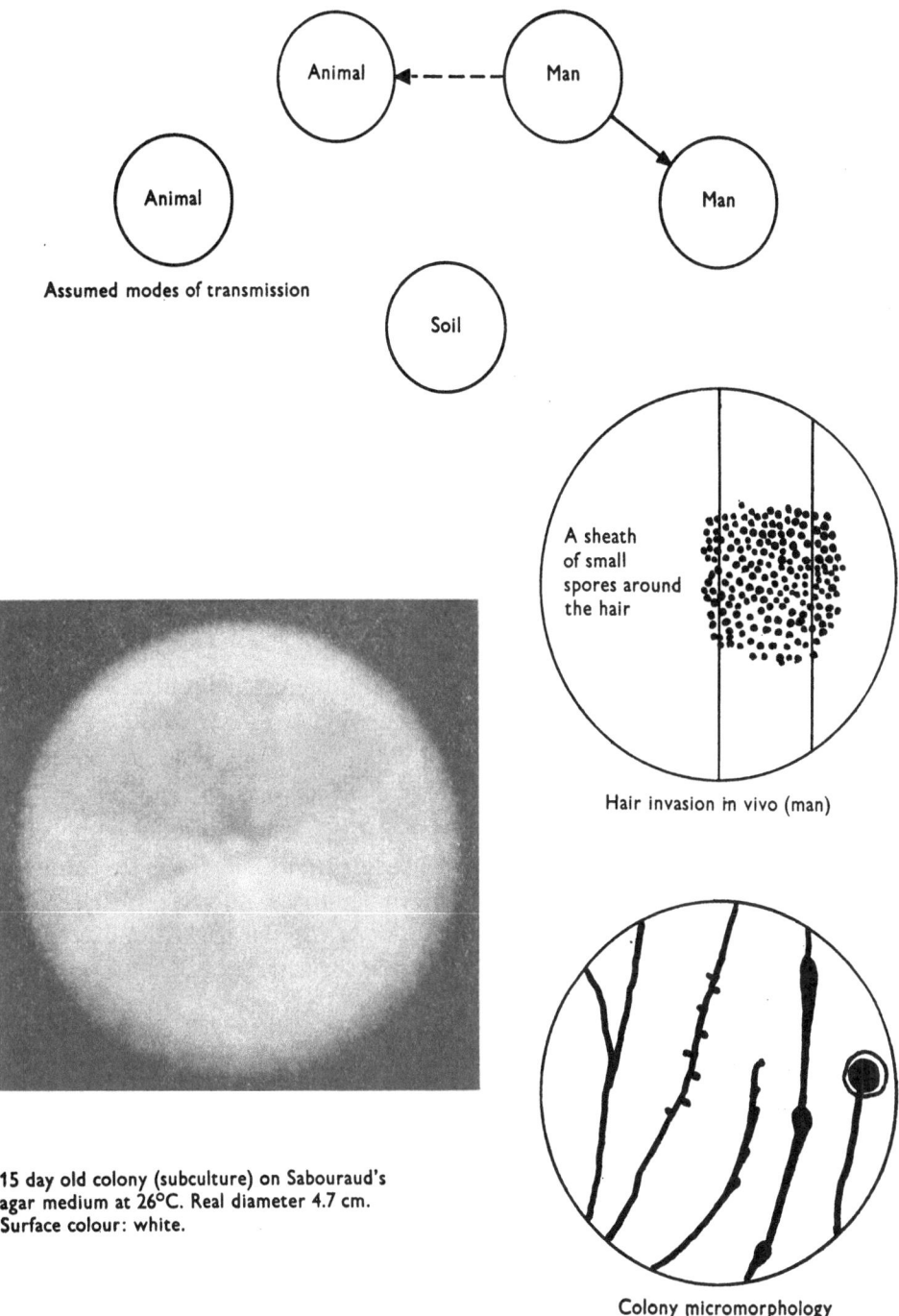

Animal

Man

Animal

Man

Assumed modes of transmission

Soil

A sheath
of small
spores around
the hair

Hair invasion in vivo (man)

15 day old colony (subculture) on Sabouraud's
agar medium at 26°C. Real diameter 4.7 cm.
Surface colour: white.

Colony micromorphology

Fig. 25. *Microsporon audouinii* Gruby 1843. World wide registered dermatophyte,
frequently attacking man and occasionally infecting animals.

Experimental pathogenicity

Pathogenicity for laboratory animals is low. Many strains were found completely incapable to cause lesions.

Nutritional requirements

Grows poorly on rice grains.

Trichophyton megninii **Blanchard, 1896**

Perfect state: not known.

Synonyms: *Trichophyton rosaceum* Sabouraud apud Bodin, 1902; *Sabouraudites megninii*
Ota et Langeron, 1923.

Some authors placed to it *Trichophyton gallinae* (e.g. CONANT et al.
1954). According to SILVA and BENHAM (1952), it must be separated as a valid
species, which can be clearly differentiated from *Trichophyton megninii*.
Trichophyton kuryangei Vanbreuseghem et Rosenthal, 1961 is considered
by VARSAVSKY and AJELLO (1964) to be a synonym of *T. megninii*.

Distribution

Saprophytic habitat and source of infection unknown. DVOŘÁK and OTČENÁŠEK
(1964) record a list of hosts of this fungus. Infection, although not too common,
is well known in some European and African countries. Animal infection seems
rare, probably of human origin. In man, tinea capitis, barbae and corporis,
exceptionally unguium, are reported. The hair invasion is of the endoectothrix
type.

Colony macromorphology

The colony attains 20—40 mm in diameter after 10 days. The mature colony
(after 15 days) has mostly a regular circular or asteroid, sometimes polygonal
ground plan. It is velvety and flat with some radial or irregular furrows and
folds. In older cultures, cracks may appear. The surface colour can be snow
white, pale rosy, vinaceous, reddish, salmon, pale lemon yellow, lilac, pale
purplish or mallow purple. The reverse is dark blood red, colcothar, rusty
or sienna. Pigment not diffusing into the environment.

Colony micromorphology

The macroconidia are normally absent or few. Some strains produce them
in limited numbers. They are clavate, slightly clavate to cigar-shaped with

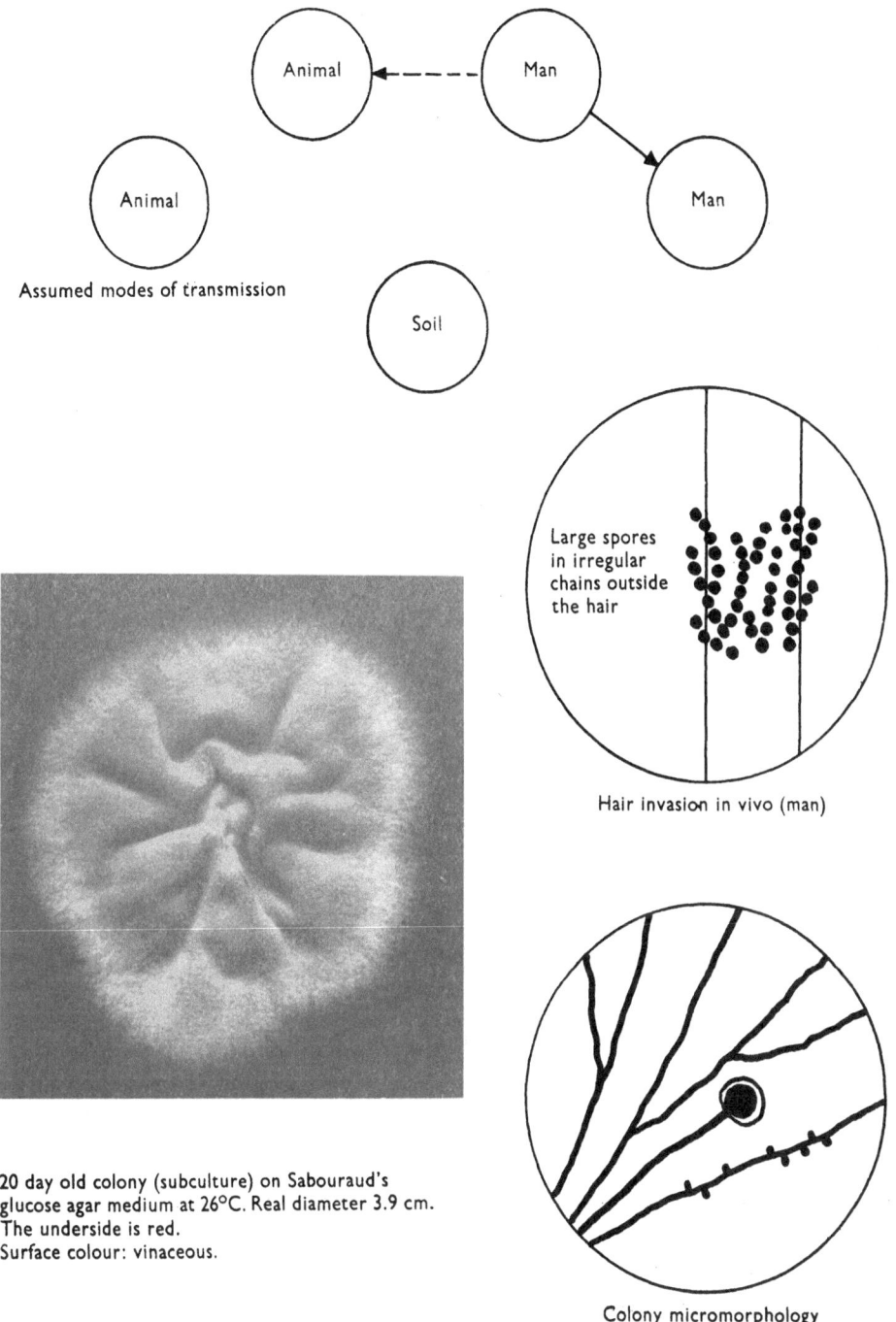

Animal

Man

Animal

Man

Assumed modes of transmission

Soil

Large spores
in irregular
chains outside
the hair

Hair invasion in vivo (man)

20 day old colony (subculture) on Sabouraud's
glucose agar medium at 26°C. Real diameter 3.9 cm.
The underside is red.
Surface colour: vinaceous.

Colony micromorphology

Fig. 26. *Trichophyton megninii* Blanchard 1896. Registered in Africa and Europe,
attacking mainly man.

thin walls, 2—8 cells, measuring 8—10 by 30—50 µm. Microconidia may also be absent, not too numerous or abundant; they are ovoid, clavate to pyriform, measuring 1—5 by 2—7·5 µm, produced from simple sporiferous hyphae (acladium type). Racquets are numerous, pectinate hyphae and spirals are occasionally produced.

Differential diagnosis

Sometimes, *T. megninii* must be differentiated from *T. gallinae* or *T. rubrum*.

Experimental pathogenicity

The cultures are always pathogenic for guinea-pigs. Erythematosquamous lesions develop after 10 days. Hair invasion of the endothrix type.

Nutritional requirements

Complete requirement for l-histidin.

Trichophyton rubrum (Castellani) Sabouraud, 1911

Perfect state: not known.

Synonyms: *Epidermophyton rubrum* Castellani, 1910; *Trichophyton purpureum* Bang, 1910.

Distribution

Saprophytic habitat and source of infection unknown. Probably mainly inter-human propagation. Human infection distributed throughout the world, very common or dominant in most countries. Known as inhabitant of the inter-digital spaces of feet, or as the cause of tinea pedis, manus, cruris, corporis and unguium, rarely of tinea capitis and barbae. Hair invasion of the endothrix or endoectothrix, large spore type. Animal infection occasional, probably of human origin. No fluorescence of infected hairs.

 DVOŘÁK and OTČENÁŠEK (1964) record a list of animal hosts of this fungus identified up to the present: cat, cattle, dog, guinea-pig, mouse, rabbit and sheep. Recently, the infection of the monkey has been reported. OTČENÁŠEK, DVOŘÁK and LADZIANSKÁ (1967) described a *T. rubrum* – like dermatophyte as the agent causing dermatophytosis in the chimpanzee.

Colony macromorphology

The colony attains 15—30 mm in diameter at the end of 10 days. The mature colony (after 10 days) has a mostly regular, circular ground plan, is fluffy,

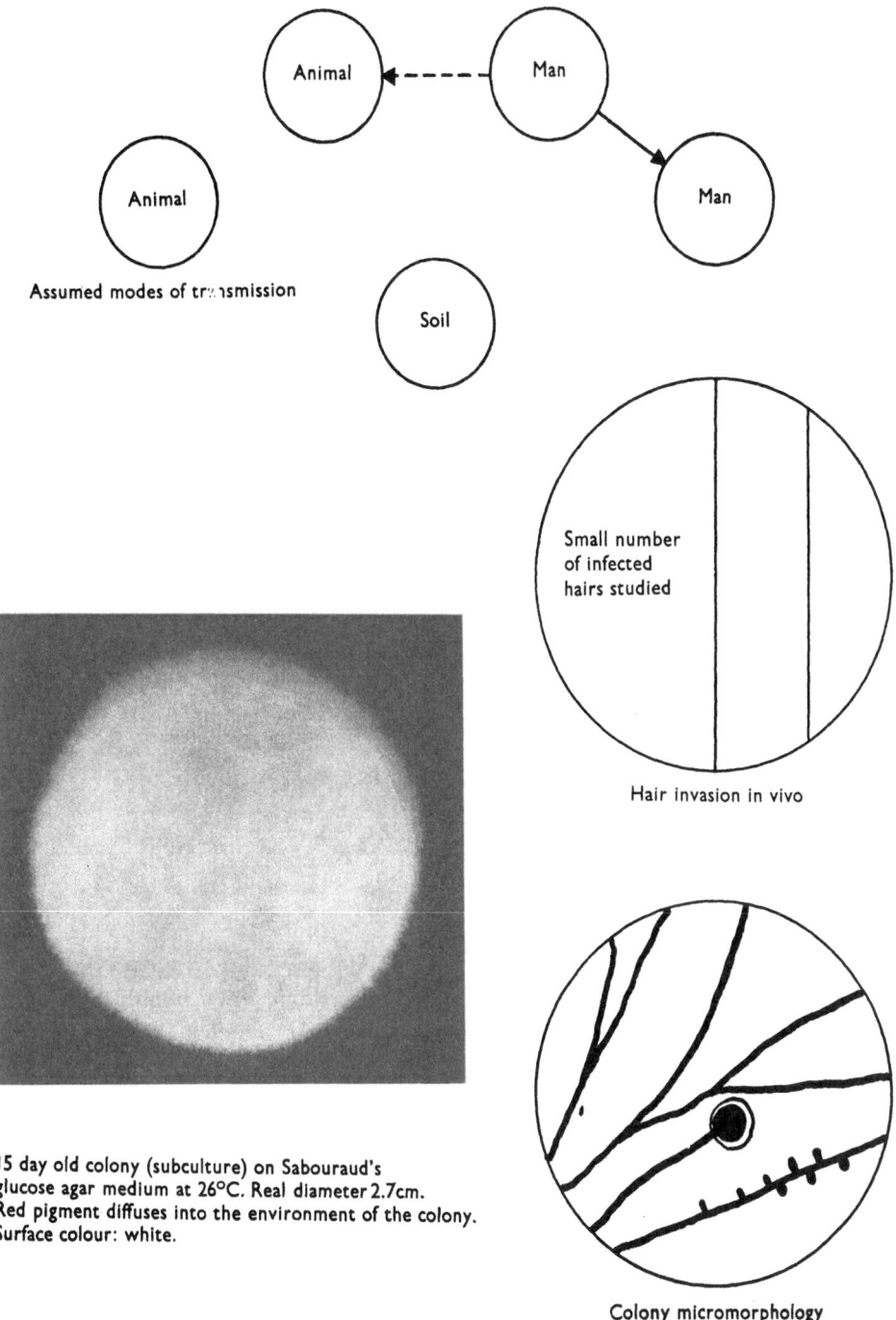

Assumed modes of transmission

Small number
of infected
hairs studied

Hair invasion in vivo

15 day old colony (subculture) on Sabouraud's
glucose agar medium at 26°C. Real diameter 2.7cm.
Red pigment diffuses into the environment of the colony.
Surface colour: white.

Colony micromorphology

Fig. 27. *Trichophyton rubrum* (Castellani) Sabouraud 1911. World wide registered
dermatophyte, frequently attacking man and occasionally infecting animals.

sometimes with a peripheral membranous zone. Occasionally, velvety or powdery strains with high folds have been observed. If the surface is formed by the endings of high aerial mycelium, no folds are seen. Mostly, the colour of the surface is snow white, only sometimes it is pale rose, rose, vinaceous, salmon, pale lemon yellow, lilac or mallow purple. At first, the colour of the velvety or granular strains is cream, later deep rose. Vinaceous diffusible pigment is produced. The reverse is carmine, dark blood red, colcothar, sometimes dark olivaceous. Sometimes, pigmentation may be absent or is yellowish orange. In some instances, the red pigmentation disappears in sub-cultures.

Colony micromorphology

The micromorphology of fluffy strains is mostly poor — only branching hyphae are found. Macroconidia in limited or abundant numbers are found only in strains with a granular surface; they are clavate to cigar-shaped, smooth, with thin walls, 3—11 cells, measuring 4—8 by 30—60 μm. Also microconidia are either absent or limited in numbers, abundant only in granular strains. They are spherical, mostly ovoid, clavate to pyriform, measuring 1—3·5 by 5—8 μm. Racquets and chlamydospores are observed; nodular bodies, pectinate hyphae or spirals occur only exceptionally.

Differential diagnosis

T. rubrum must be differentiated from *T. gallinae*, *T. megninii* and *T. mentagrophytes* var. *interdigitale*.

Experimental pathogenicity

Some strains are nonpathogenic. With some strains, experimental infection of guinea-pigs has been successful. Hair invasion of the endoectothrix type.

Keratinolysis of hairs in vitro

T. rubrum attacks coaxially the hairs of cattle, dog, goat, horse, mouse and man.

Nutritional requirement

No special requirements.

Trichophyton schoenleinii (Lebert) **Langeron et Milochevitch, 1930**

Perfect state: not known.

Synonyms: *Oidium schoenleinii* Lebert, 1843; *Achorion schoenleinii* Remak, 1845.

Some authors place to it *Trichophyton verrucosum* (e.g. CONANT et al. 1945). AINSWORTH and GEORG (1945) separated *Trichophyton verrucosum* as a valid species with 4 varieties.

Distribution

Saprophytic habitat and source of infection unknown. A single isolation from garden soil has been recorded (ref. COUDERT, BATTESTI and MICHEL-BRUN 1966), which seemed to have survived there without reproduction. Mainly interhuman propagation probable. Human infection of world wide distribution, in some countries most frequent. Known as the cause of human favus with the possibility of developing into a severe generalized infection. Mostly tinea capitis and corporis reported. The hair is penetrated by hyphae and a scutulum consisting of hyphae and spores is formed round its base. No fluorescence of infected hairs. Animal infection seems to be accidental, probably of human origin. DVOŘÁK and OTČENÁŠEK (1964) record a list of animal hosts of this fungus, identified up to the present: bird (unknown species), cat, cattle, dog, guinea-pig, horse, mouse, rabbit.

Colony macromorphology

The colony grows slowly, attaining a diameter of 10—20 mm after 10 days. The nature colony (after 20 days) may have a regular to asteroid ground plan or may be irregularly asteroid, polygonal or lobulate. Mostly, it is membranous, sometimes entirely glabrous, sometimes with a short, more or less dense, velvety or slightly powdered mycelium, always wrinkled to some extent. Occasional strains grow largely submerged in the agar. The surface colour may be gray to tan, salmon, pale lemon yellow or pale yellow greenish. Sometimes brownish, diffusing pigment is observed. The reverse without pigmentation or of pale lemon yellow colour.

Colony micromorphology

The micromorphology is poor — typical macroconidia are seldom observed. In some cases, a few irregular, smooth macroconidia with thin walls, 5—11 cells, measuring 6—11 by 35—85 μm, are found. Typical microconidia are not produced, sometimes their production is mimicked by small chlamydospores. Typical is the presence of numerous favic chandeliers in some strains. Pectinate hyphae are rare whereas chlamydospores are abundant.

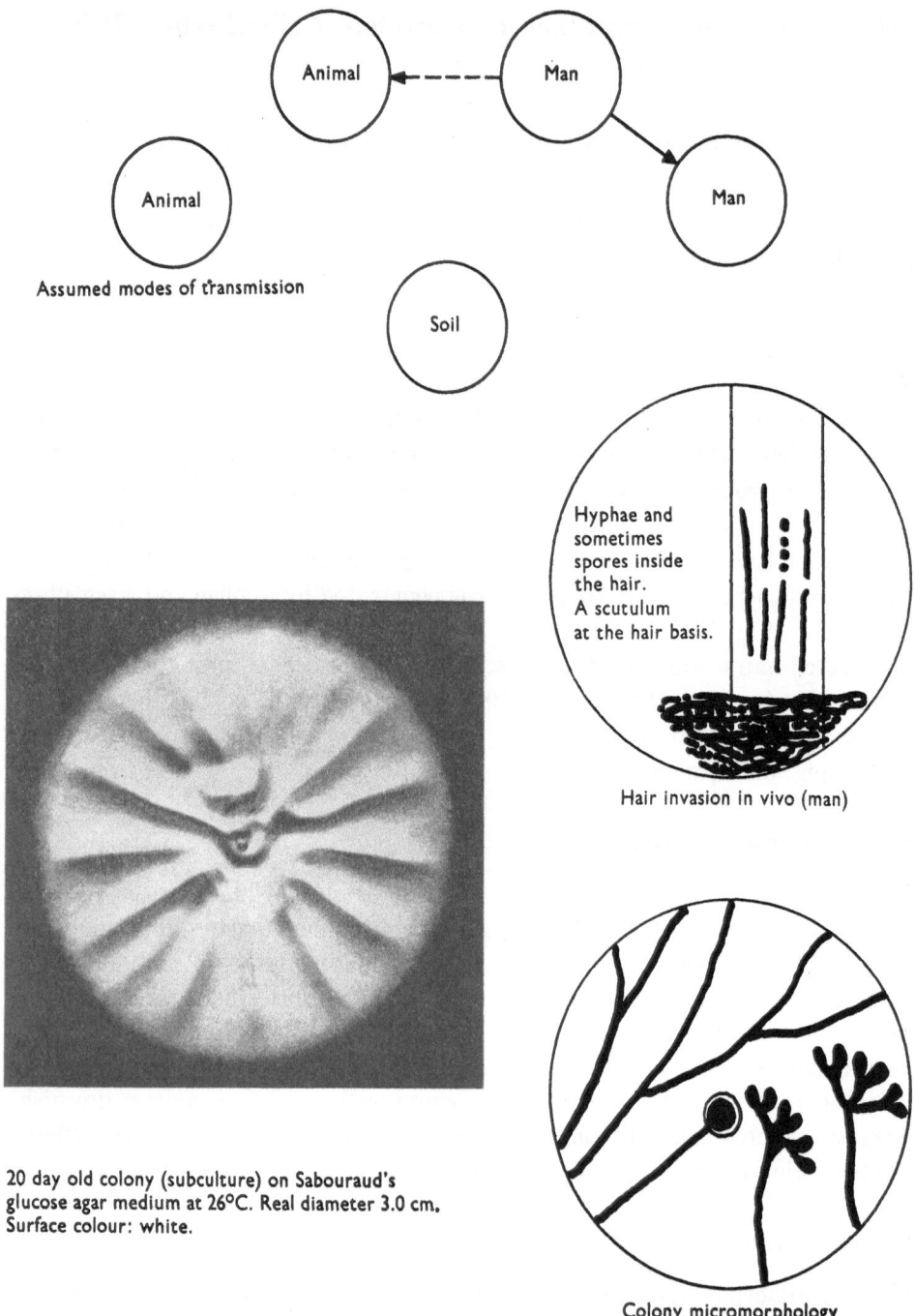

Assumed modes of transmission

Hyphae and sometimes spores inside the hair. A scutulum at the hair basis.

Hair invasion in vivo (man)

20 day old colony (subculture) on Sabouraud's glucose agar medium at 26°C. Real diameter 3.0 cm. Surface colour: white.

Colony micromorphology

Fig. 28. *Trichophyton schoenleinii* (Lebert) Langeron et Milochevitch 1930. World wide registered dermatophyte, frequently attacking man and occasionally infecting animals.

Differential diagnosis

T. schoenleinii must sometimes be differentiated from *T. concentricum* and *T. verrucosum*.

Experimental pathogenicity

A wide range of animals has been successfully inoculated. Pathogenic for the guinea-pig.

Nutritional requirements

No special requirements.

Trichophyton tonsurans Malmsten, 1845

Perfect state: not known.

Synonyms: *Trichophyton epilans* Mégnin, 1890; *Trichophyton sabouraudii* Blanchard, 1896; *Trichophyton acuminatum* Bodin, 1902; *Trichophyton crateriforme* Bodin, 1902; *Trichophyton cerebriforme* Sabouraud, 1910.

For *Trichophyton tonsurans* Malmsten var. *sulphureum* Sabouraud, 1910 or *Trichophyton sulphureum* Fox, 1908 see p. 138.

CONANT et al. (1954) differentiated the following species: *T. epilans* (syn. e.g. *T. cerebriforme*), *T. tonsurans* (syn. e.g. *T. crateriforme*), *T. sabouraudii* (syn. e.g. *T. acuminatum*) and *T. sulphureum*.

Distribution

Saprophytic habitat and source of infection unknown. Probably mainly inter-human propagation. Human infection of world wide distribution, frequent in some countries. Known especially as the cause of tinea capitis, corporis and barbae, rarely even as the cause of tinea pedis and unguium. Hair invasion of the endothrix type. No fluorescence of the infected hairs. Animal infection (horse) seems to be sporadic and probably of human origin. Its resemblance to *T. equinum* merits attention. It seems, however, that *T. tonsurans* is still common in countries, where horses are propagated on a larger scale. In Czechoslovakia, where the number of horses has dropped down considerably in recent years, *T. tonsurans*, previously most common in this country, is now practically nonexistant.

Colony macromorphology

The colony attains a diameter of 10—30 mm after 10 days. The mature colony (after 10 days) has a regular, circular to asteroid ground plan, which may

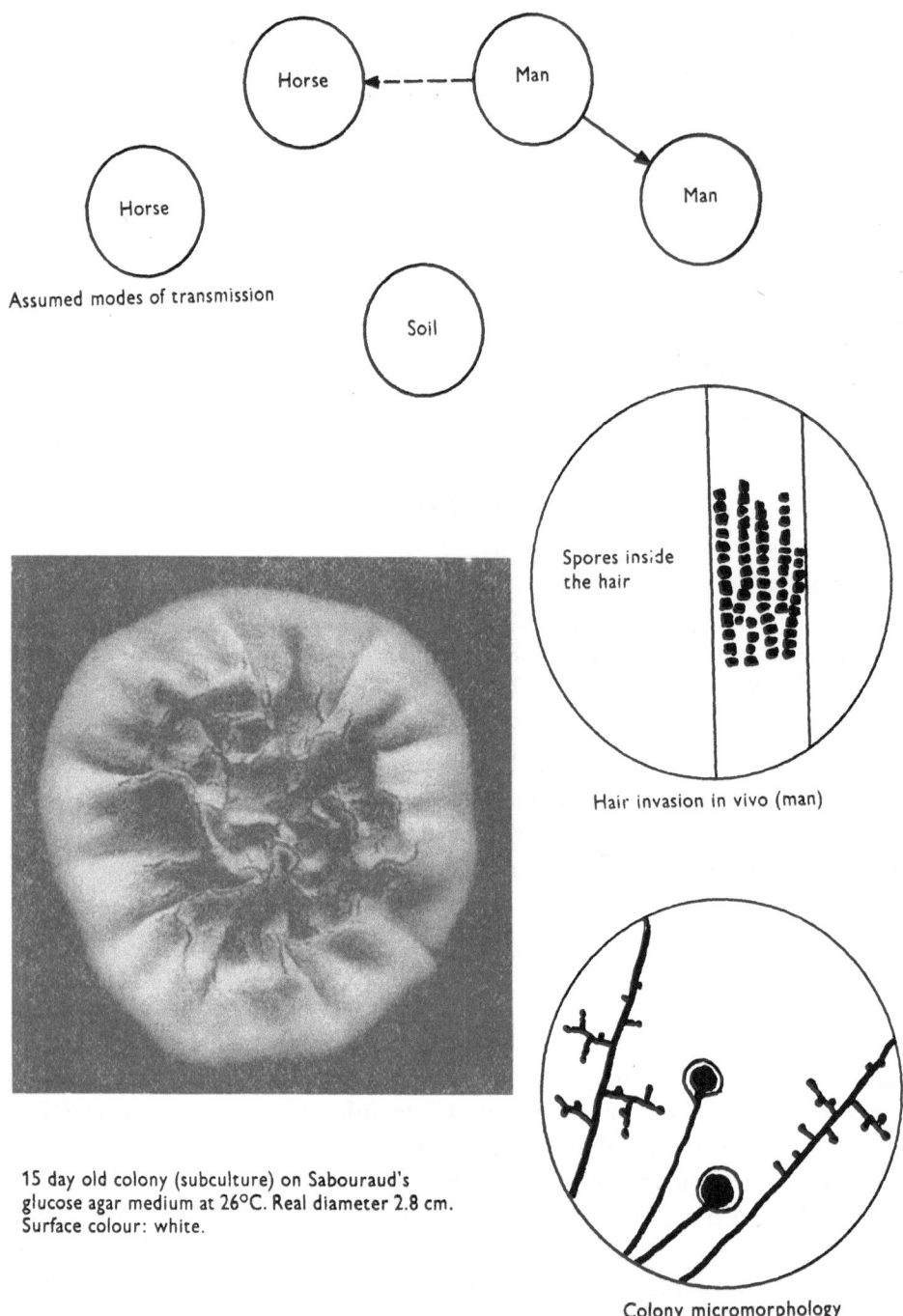

Horse ← - - - Man → Man

Horse

Soil

Assumed modes of transmission

Spores inside the hair

Hair invasion in vivo (man)

15 day old colony (subculture) on Sabouraud's glucose agar medium at 26°C. Real diameter 2.8 cm. Surface colour: white.

Colony micromorphology

Fig. 29. *Trichophyton tonsurans* Malmsten 1845. World wide registered dermatophyte, commonly attacking man.

sometimes be also irregularly polygonal. It is typical for the colonies to be at first finely granular, later sometimes velvety powdered, flat at the beginning, then more or less wrinkled. The surface colour is cream to tan, but can also be gray, rosy, salmon, pale lemon yellow, lemon yellow, sometimes brownish. The reverse is saffron yellow, mahagony red to brownish.

Colony micromorphology

In some strains no macroconidia are found, in others they are present in limited numbers. They are clavate to spindle-shaped, smooth, thin, with 2—10 cells, measuring 4—12 by 20—80 µm. Microconidia are always numerous, produced en thyrses (acladium type) and en grappe (botrytis type). They are ovoid, clavate to pyriform, measuring 2—3·5 by 4·5—10 µm. Pectinate hyphae and racquets may be present, chlamydospores are abundant.

Differential diagnosis

T. tonsurans must sometimes be differentiated from *T. equinum* and *T. mentagrophytes*.

Experimental pathogenicity

Pathogenic for the guinea-pig.

Nutritional requirements

Grows poorly on casein media.

Trichophyton violaceum Sabouraud apud Bodin, 1902

Perfect state: not known.

Synonyms: *Trichophyton glabrum* Sabouraud, 1910; *Achorion violaceum* Bloch, 1911; *Sabouraudites violaceus* Ota et Langeron, 1923.

Some authors placed to it also *Trichophyton gourvilii* Catanei, 1933 (e.g. CONANT et al. 1954). Recently, *T. gourvilii* has been considered to be a valid species (e.g. VARSAVSKY and AJELLO 1964).

Distribution

Saprophytic habitat and source of infection unknown. Probably mainly inter-human propagation. Human infection world wide, very frequent in some

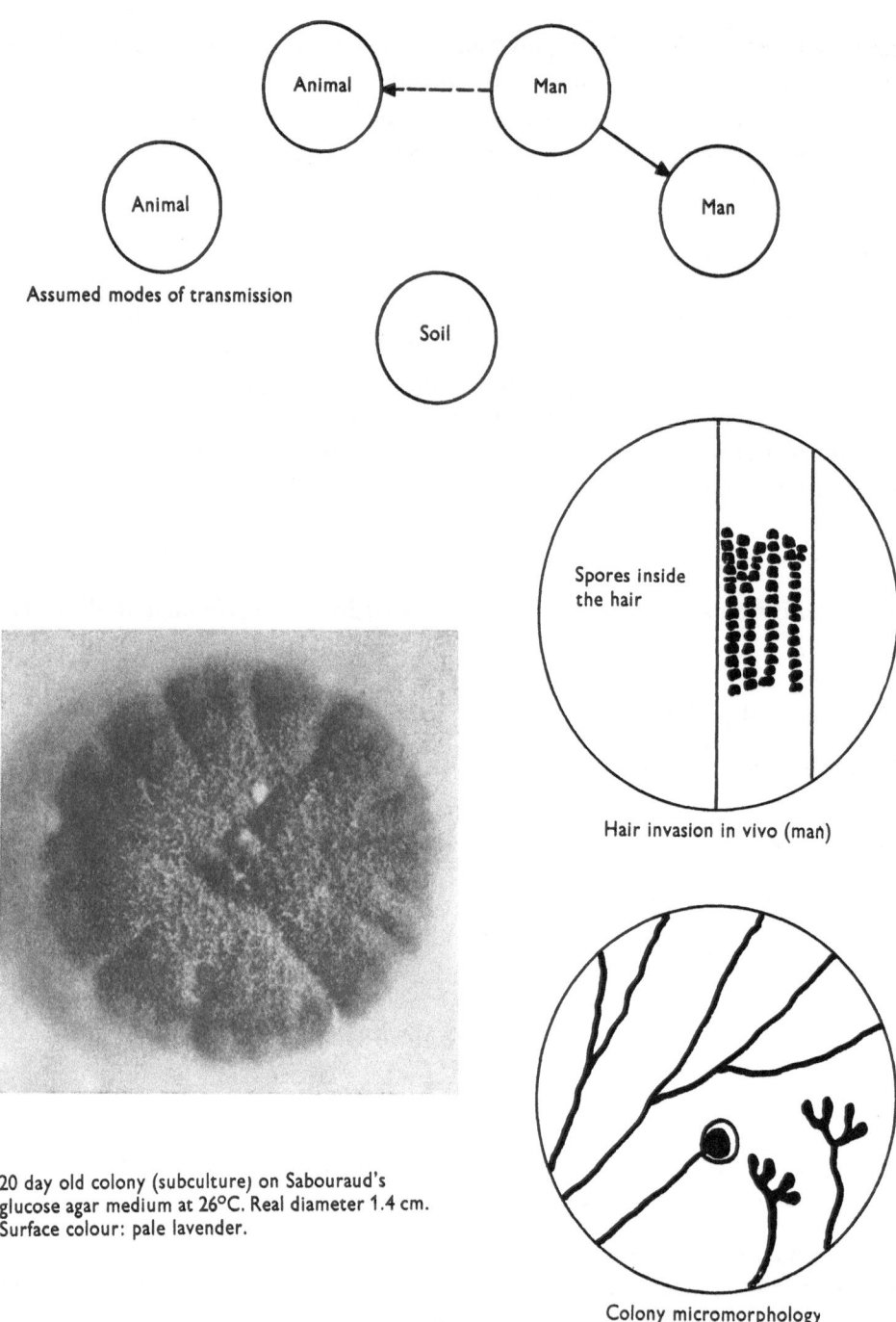

Assumed modes of transmission

Spores inside
the hair

Hair invasion in vivo (man)

20 day old colony (subculture) on Sabouraud's
glucose agar medium at 26°C. Real diameter 1.4 cm.
Surface colour: pale lavender.

Colony micromorphology

Fig. 30. *Trichophyton violaceum* Sabouraud apud Bodin 1902. World wide registered
dermatophyte, frequently attacking man and occasionally infecting animals.

countries. Known especially as the cause of tinea capitis and corporis, but also of tinea barbae and unguium. Sometimes the lesions are favus-like. Hair invasion of the endothrix type. No fluorescence of the infected hairs. Animal infection sporadic, probably of human origin. DVOŘÁK and OTČENÁŠEK (1964) record a list of animal hosts of this fungus, identified up to the present: cat, cattle, dog, horse, mouse, pigeon. Recently, an infection of buffaloes has been recorded (REFAI 1966).

Colony macromorphology

The colony grows slowly, attaining a diameter of 5—15 mm after 10 days. The mature colony (after 20 days) may have a regular — circular to asteroid — or irregular — polygonal to lobulate ground plan. It is typical for the surface to be entirely membranous, glabrous, humid, sometimes slightly powdered. The colony is always more or less wrinkled or verrucose. The surface colour can be gray or cream, dark blood red, salmon, pale violaceous, pale lavender, lavender violaceous, violet, purplish, purple, dark purple, livid purple, purplish gray or purplish black. The reverse colour is in accord with the surface pigmentation.

Colony micromorphology

The micromorphology is poor. Mostly only slender branching hyphae are found. Macroconidia are absent in almost all strains. Exceptionally, strains are found which produce several irregular, smooth macroconidia with thin walls, 2—8 cells, measuring 4—6 by 30—40 µm. Normally, microconidia are also absent and only some strains produce them in limited numbers. They are ovoid, clavate to pyriform, 2—3 by 3—4 µm. Sometimes, favic chandeliers and pectinate hyphae are found.

Differential diagnosis

T. violaceum must sometimes be differentiated from *T. yaoundei*.

Experimental pathogenicity

Pathogenic for guinea-pigs.

Nutritional requirements

Grows poorly on casein media.

Geophilic dermatophytes attacking or contaminating animals and man

With the exception of *M. cookei* and *M. nanum*, which we have not been able to isolate until now, we have studied the properties of all other dermatophytes of this group on numerous strains obtained from soil (e.g. Dvořák, Přikryl and Sobota 1959, Otčenášek, Dvořák and Silva Taboada 1965), from the hairs of apparently healthy animals (Otčenášek and Dvořák 1962) and on several strains of *M. gypseum* isolated from human lesions.

It is possible that also *M. vanbreuseghemii* belongs to the geophilic, primarily soil saprophytizing species, but all attempts of isolating it from soil have failed. *M. cookei* had to be studied only in subculture of our collection. Recently, *M. fulvum* was separated from *M. gypseum* and therefore, it is not possible to outline their properties separately.

Keratinomyces ajelloi Vanbreuseghem, 1952

Perfect state: *Arthroderma uncinatum* Dawson et Gentles, 1961,
   Anixiopsis stercoraria (Hansen) Hansen, 1893*.
Variety: *K. ajelloi* Vanbreuseghem var. *nana* Hejtmánek et Kunert, 1965.

Distribution

Terrestrial dermatophyte of world wide distribution, common in some countries and absent in others. In Czechoslovakia, this dermatophyte was first isolated by Dvořák in 1955—1956, who identified it as a fungus similar to *M. gypseum* (ref. Hejtmánek 1957). Later e.g. Hejtmánek (1957), Dvořák, Přikryl and Sobota (1959) recorded its repeated isolation. In Cuba, after careful studies of about 200 soil samples from various regions, only *M. gypseum* and *T. terrestre* were isolated (Dvořák, Otčenášek and Silva Taboada 1965, Otčenášek, Dvořák and Silva Taboada 1965). Dvořák and Otčenášek (1964) record a list of occasional hosts of this dermatophyte, which they found

---

* Single report by Benedek (1963).

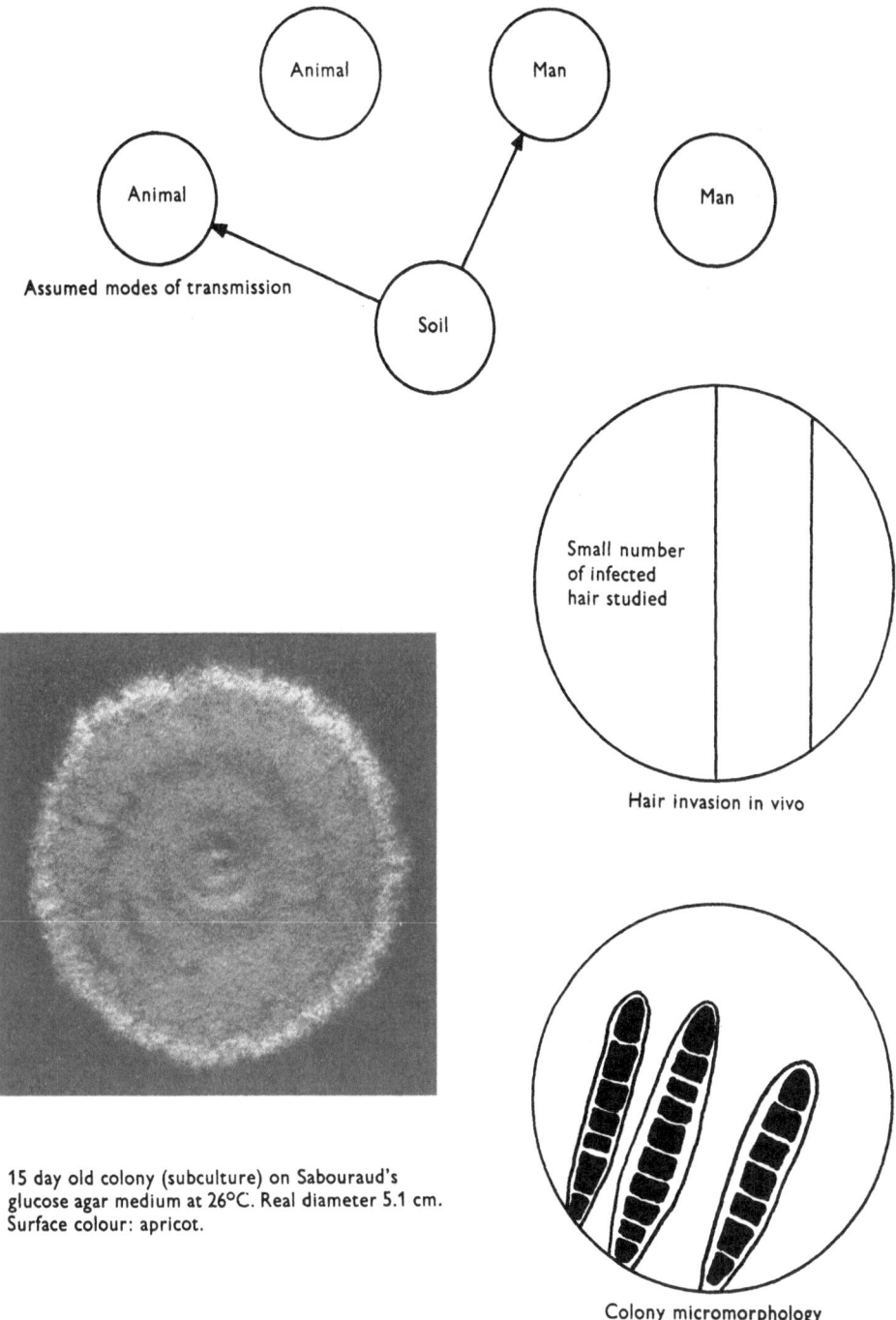

Assumed modes of transmission

Small number
of infected
hair studied

Hair invasion in vivo

15 day old colony (subculture) on Sabouraud's
glucose agar medium at 26°C. Real diameter 5.1 cm.
Surface colour: apricot.

Colony micromorphology

Fig. 31. *Keratinomyces ajelloi* Vanbreuseghem 1952. World wide distributed dermatophyte, occurring in soil, occasionally attacking man and animals.

in lesions probably caused by it: cattle, dog, guinea-pig, horse and man. In the latter, tinea corporis has been recorded. Similar infection, caused by *M. gypseum*, is probably of soil origin. Hair invasion of the endothrix type. No fluorescence of infected hairs.

Colony macromorphology

The colony attains a diameter of 15—40 mm after 10 days. The mature colony (after 10 days) has mostly a regular ground plan — circular to asteroid. The surface is granular, sometimes velvety powdered, entirely flat or with some radial, shallow furrows. The surface colour is cream, tan to orange tan, but also salmon, apricot, saffron yellow, orange or pale lemon yellow. The reverse is apricot, saffron yellow, sepia or lemon yellow, sometimes purplish black or bluish black; diffusible pigment is produced. Some strains are colourless. "Pleomorphic degeneration" may soon appear.

Colony micromorphology

The most important diagnostic sign is the presence of numerous cigar-shaped to spindle-shaped smooth macroconidia with thick walls, 4—24 cells, measuring 8—19 by 16—40 μm. Our strains produced a few ovoid, clavate to pyriform microconidia (3—7 by 5—13 μm), sessile, mostly borne en thyrses (acladium type). Nodular bodies, pectinate hyphae, racquets and spirals may be present. Especially in older culture, chlamydospores may be abundant.

Differential diagnosis

Sometimes, this dermatophyte must be differentiated from *M. vanbreuseghemii*.

Experimental pathogenicity

Inoculation of most strains isolated was unsuccessful. Some strains are capable of producing lesions in the guinea-pig.

Keratinolysis of hairs in vitro

K. ajelloi attacks rectangularly the hairs of man, coaxially the hairs of the dog, goat, horse and man, both rectangularly and coaxially the hairs of cattle.

Nutritional requirements

No special requirements

Perfect state (*Arthroderma uncinatum*):

Cleistothecia: size 300—900 μm.
Colour: buff.

Character of peridium: terminal branches of hyphae usually with more than three cells; cell dumbbell-shaped, strongly constricted, mostly symmetrical.

Peridial appendages — spirals of different length.

Keratinomyces ajelloi Vanbreuseghem var. *nana* Hejtmánek and Kunert, 1965

Isolated from soil in the vicinity of Olomouc (KUNERT and HEJTMÁNEK 1964). It is considered to be a stable morphological mutant differing from *K. ajelloi* particularly in visibly shortened macroconidia.

The colony attains a diameter of approximately 20 mm after 10 days. The mature colony (after 10 days) is granular and flat. Its margin is white, its central part saffron yellow. The reverse is brownish — the pigment is not diffusing into the medium. The most important diagnostic sign is the presence of numerous spindle-shaped to clavate, smooth macroconidia with thick walls, 1—7 cells, measuring 7—19 by 16—40 µm. Also pyriform microconidia of 3—5 by 3—6 µm are found. Spirals and chlamydospores are produced. The culture has been found to be apathogenic.

Microsporon cookei Ajello, 1959

Perfect state: *Nannizzia cajetana* Ajello, 1961.

This fungus was isolated from soil by Cooke in the U.S.A. Emm soil identified it as a variety of *M. gypseum* (see AJELLO 1959). AJELLO (1959) isolated it from soil and from the skin of various apparently healthy animals and described it as a new species. Later, it was isolated from lesions in a dog (AJELLO 1959), in a cat (JAKSCH and THURNER 1966), a baboon (MARIAT and TAPIA 1966), a guinea-pig and man (ŠIK 1965).

Distribution

This geophilic dermatophyte seems to contaminate frequently the skin and to attack occasionally animals and man. In the latter the infection is evidently of soil origin. *M. cookei* seems to be distributed throughout the world, although it has not been recorded from some countries until now. In Czechoslovakia, it was first isolated by HEJTMÁNEK (1962).

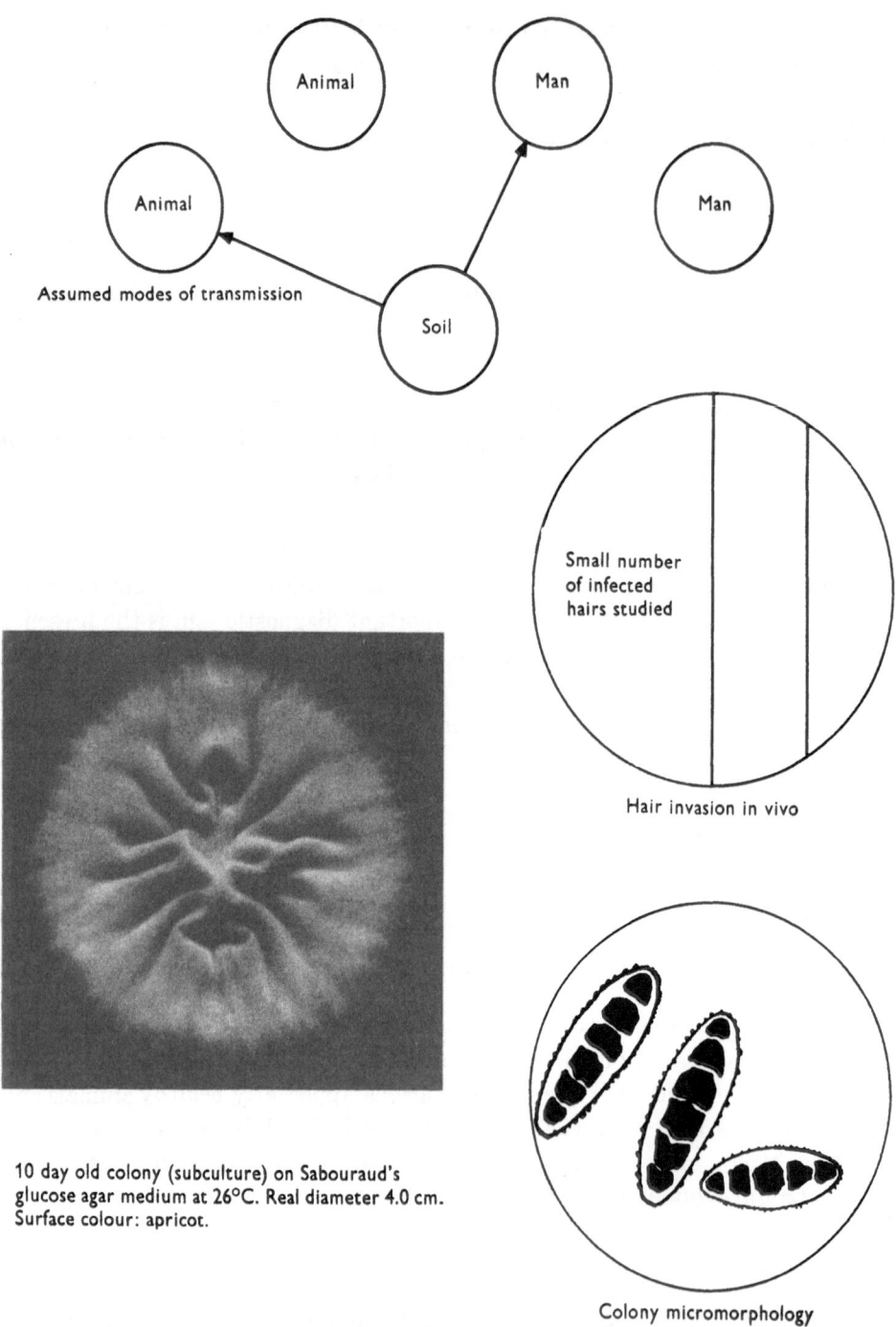

Assumed modes of transmission

Small number of infected hairs studied

Hair invasion in vivo

10 day old colony (subculture) on Sabouraud's glucose agar medium at 26°C. Real diameter 4.0 cm. Surface colour: apricot.

Colony micromorphology

Fig. 32. *Microsporon cookei* Ajello 1959. Dermatophyte occurring in soil, occasionally attacking man and animals.

Colony macromorphology

The colony attains a diameter of 10—40 mm after 10 days. The mature colony has mostly a regular ground plan — circular to asteroid. It is granular to velvety powdered, sometimes with a relatively large portion of submerged periphery. The surface can be entirely flat or with some radial, shallow furrows. Its colour is pale rosy, rosy, salmon, apricot, pale lemon yellow to lilac. Sometimes, a white velvety margin is observed. The reverse can be dark blood red, orange, rusty to olivaceous. Diffusible pigment, when produced, is mostly lemon yellow and can be viewed at the periphery of the colony. "Pleomorphic degeneration" has been observed.

Colony micromorphology

The most important diagnostic sign is the presence of numerous spindle-shaped rough macroconidia with thick walls, 6—10 cells, measuring 12—28 by 31 to 75 μm. Microconidia are mostly found in limited numbers. They are ovoid, clavate to pyriform, measuring 2—4 by 3—8 μm; also spirals have been observed.

Experimental pathogenicity

Most strains seem to be apathogenic for guinea-pig and rabbit although some strains seem to be capable of producing lesions in guinea-pigs.

Nutritional requirements

No special requirements.

Perfect state (*Nannizzia cajetana*):

Cleistothecium: size 400—700 μm.
Colour: light brown.
Character of peridium: hyphae radial, often branched in verticillate manner, hyphal cells cylindrical without constriction. Peridial appendages — spirals of different length, tapered hyphae.

Microsporon gypseum (Bodin) Guiart et Grigorakis, 1928

Perfect states: *Nannizzia gypsea* (Nannizzi) Stockdale, 1963,
    Nannizzia incurvata Stockdale, 1961.

Recently, *M. fulvum* Uriburu, 1909 has been separated and its perfect state (*Nannizzia fulva* Stockdale, 1963) discovered. Until STOCKDALE (1963) re-established *M. fulvum*, this species was not recorded and only sporadically its original description was given. Therefore, we have made only a description of the *M. gypseum* "complex". The separation of *M. fulvum* makes it necessary to revise some data and to study a number of strains from this new aspect.

Distribution

Terrestrial, world wide distributed dermatophyte, very common in some countries, absent in others. DVOŘÁK and OTČENÁŠEK (1964) record a list of animal hosts of this dermatophyte: cat, daman, dog, donkey, guinea-pig, horse, monkey, mouse, rabbit, rat, swine, tiger and chicken. Recently, ringworm caused by it has been identified in the buffalo and the tapir (REFAI 1966). *M. gypseum* infection of animals and man is not so scarce as infection caused by other geophilic dermatophytes. Animal infection appears to be more common than human infection (GEORG 1960), but it is impossible to give reliable information on the relative frequency of this infection. In eastern Bohemia, dermatophytic lesions of 627 potential hosts of this fungus were examined in 1962—1964. Results were negative (DVOŘÁK, OTČENÁŠEK and KOMÁREK 1965). Up to 1966, we have not identified this fungus as an animal parasite, although we found it most frequently in Czechoslovak soil. In view of the results of our examinations from the last decade, *M. gypseum* causes dermatophytic lesions in about 1% of cases. Also infection of man seems to be of soil origin. The anamnesis of most patients points to close contact with soil (e.g. gardeners). In man, tinea capitis and corporis have been observed most frequently; tinea barbae, pedis and unguium are exceptional. Hair invasion of the endoectothrix type (large spores of 5—8 μm); sometimes, favus-like lesions develop. No fluorescence or very poor fluorescence of infected hairs.

Colony macromorphology

The colony attains a diameter of 25—50 mm after 10 days. The mature colony has mostly a regular ground plan, circular to asteroid. Sometimes, the colony is entirely asteroid except its small central part, consisting of rays or radial, cord-like formations. It can be entirely flat and granular. Circular, granular colonies can be velvety to fluffy in their marginal part. Some colonies are velvety powdered. There is little tendency of the colony to wrinkle and only in some strains, some shallow radial furrows are observed. The surface colour is light ochre to deep cinnamon brown or rosy, salmon, apricot or pale lemon yellow. The fluffy or velvety margin is white when formed. The reverse is dull yellow to tan, rarely pinkish to red; it can be egg-yolk yellow, apricot, orange, terracotta or pale lemon yellow. Diffusible pigment not produced. Sometimes, pleomorphic mycelium soon appears.

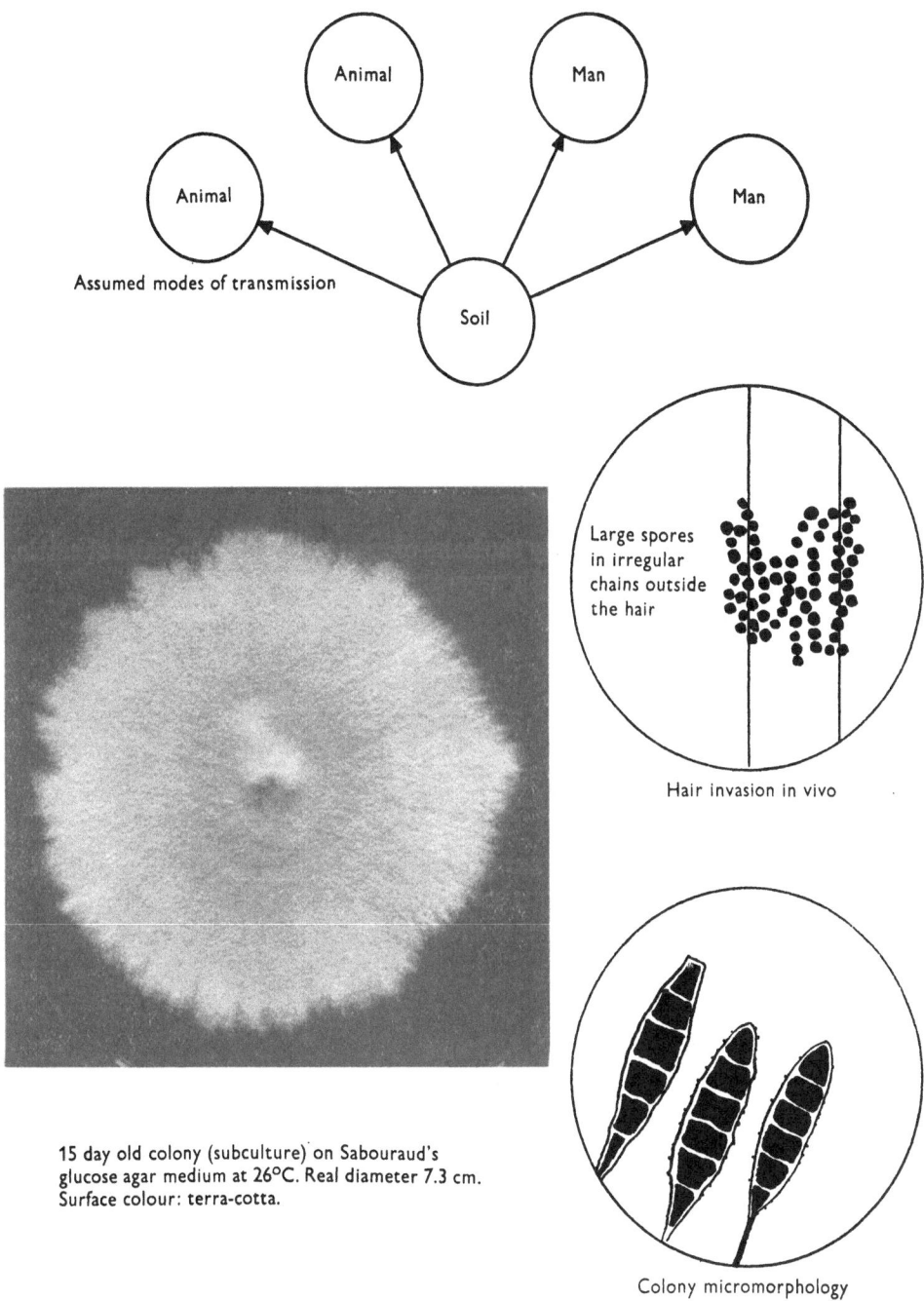

Animal   Man   Animal   Man

Assumed modes of transmission

Soil

Large spores
in irregular
chains outside
the hair

Hair invasion in vivo

15 day old colony (subculture) on Sabouraud's
glucose agar medium at 26°C. Real diameter 7.3 cm.
Surface colour: terra-cotta.

Colony micromorphology

Fig. 33. *Microsporon gypseum* (Bodin) Guiart et Grigorakis 1928. World wide distributed dermatophyte occurring in soil, attacking man and animals.

Colony micromorphology

The most important diagnostic sign is the presence of numerous spindle-shaped, rough macroconidia with thin walls, 3—9 cells, measuring 6—18 by 24—80 μm. Our strains mostly produced macroconidia of 5—6 cells. Some strains produce microconidia in limited numbers; strains producing an abundance of microconidia are quite exceptional. The microconidia are clavate (1·5—3·5 by 2·5—8·5 μm) sessile, borne en thyrses (acladium type). Nodular bodies, pectinate hyphae, racquets, spirals and chlamydospores are sporadically found.

Experimental pathogenicity

Pathogenic for many animals. Lesions can be easily produced in guinea-pigs.

Keratinolysis of hairs in vitro

M. gypseum attacks rectangularly the hairs of man, coaxially the hairs of cattle, goat, horse and mouse and in both ways the hairs of the dog.

Nutritional requirements

No special requirements.

Perfect state (*Nannizzia fulva*):

Cleistothecium: size 500—1,250 μm.
Colour: light buff.
Character of peridium: hyphae curved towards cleistothecium or radial, side by side. (For remaining signs see foregoing species.)
Peridial appendages — spirals most frequent, sometimes branched, tapered hyphae.

Perfect state (*Nannizzia gypsea*):

Cleistothecium: size 300—750 (—900) μm.
Colour: light buff.
Character of peridium: hyphae curved towards cleistothecium with up to 4 verticillate-like branches, hyphal cells with 1—3 constrictions.
Peridial appendages — spirals of different length, tapered hyphae.

Perfect state (*Nannizzia incurvata*):

Cleistothecium: size 350—650 (—900) μm.
Colour: light buff.
Character of peridium: hyphae radial, often divided into five verticillate-like branches, hyphal cells with 1—3 constrictions.
Peridial appendages — spirals of different length, tapered hyphae.

110

Microsporon nanum Fuentes, 1956

Perfect state: *Nannizzia obtusa* Dawson et Gentles, 1961.

The first isolate described as a dwarf variety of *M. gypseum* — *M. gypseum* (Bodin) Guiart et Grigorakis var. *nana* Fuentes, Aboulafia et Vidal, 1954.

Distribution

First reported from Cuba (tinea capitis) by FUENTES, ABOULAFIA and VIDAL (1954) and FUENTES (1956). DAWSON and GENTLES (1961) obtained cultures of this fungus isolated from swine in Kenya. BROCK (1961) reported the isolation of *M. nanum* from a case of tinea capitis in man in Louisiana. BUBASH, GINTHER and AJELLO (1964) report on an outbreak of this fungus infection in a herd of swine in Pennsylvania. GINTHER et al. (1964) found this dermatophyte as the cause of ringworm in swine in Kansas, Kentucky and New Jersey; DODD, NEWLIN and NIKSCH (1965) in Indiana; GINTHER (1965) based his study on the clinical aspects of *M. nanum* also on observations from Georgia, Illinois, Iowa, Maryland, Missouri, Tennessee and Texas. It has also been found in Mexico (BEIRANA and MAGANA 1960), in Canada (CARMICHAEL and REID 1961), in Australia — Queensland (CONNOLE and BAYNES 1966). Recently, *M. nanum* has been isolated from soil. There is also information on its capability of reproducing in soil. The infection seems to be mainly of soil origin, but the transmission of this fungus, especially from swine to man, should be anticipated.

Brief characteristics of the disease

Cases of infection with this dermatophyte are known to occur mostly in the adult swine, especially in the sow; reports of infection of young pigs and sucking pigs are sporadic.

Pathological changes are either diffusely distributed over the animal's body (DODD et al. 1965, GINTHER 1965), or restricted to certain areas: ear lobes, anterior and posterior extremities, abdominal region (e.g. CONNOLE and BAYNES 1966).

The skin of the attacked parts reddens, becomes uneven, but the foci are not elevated and mostly, there is no loss of hair. The foci are covered with minute, numerous brownish scales (GINTHER 1965). Some authors describe the formation of grayish brown crusts with the red background base shining through. Desquamated epithelium forms a dark peripheral zone. Alopecia and pruritus have not been recorded (CONNOLE and BAYNES 1966). According to GINTHER (1965) the affected parts have a mud-like appearance; after washing off the crusts, the dermatophytosis can be recognized only by the

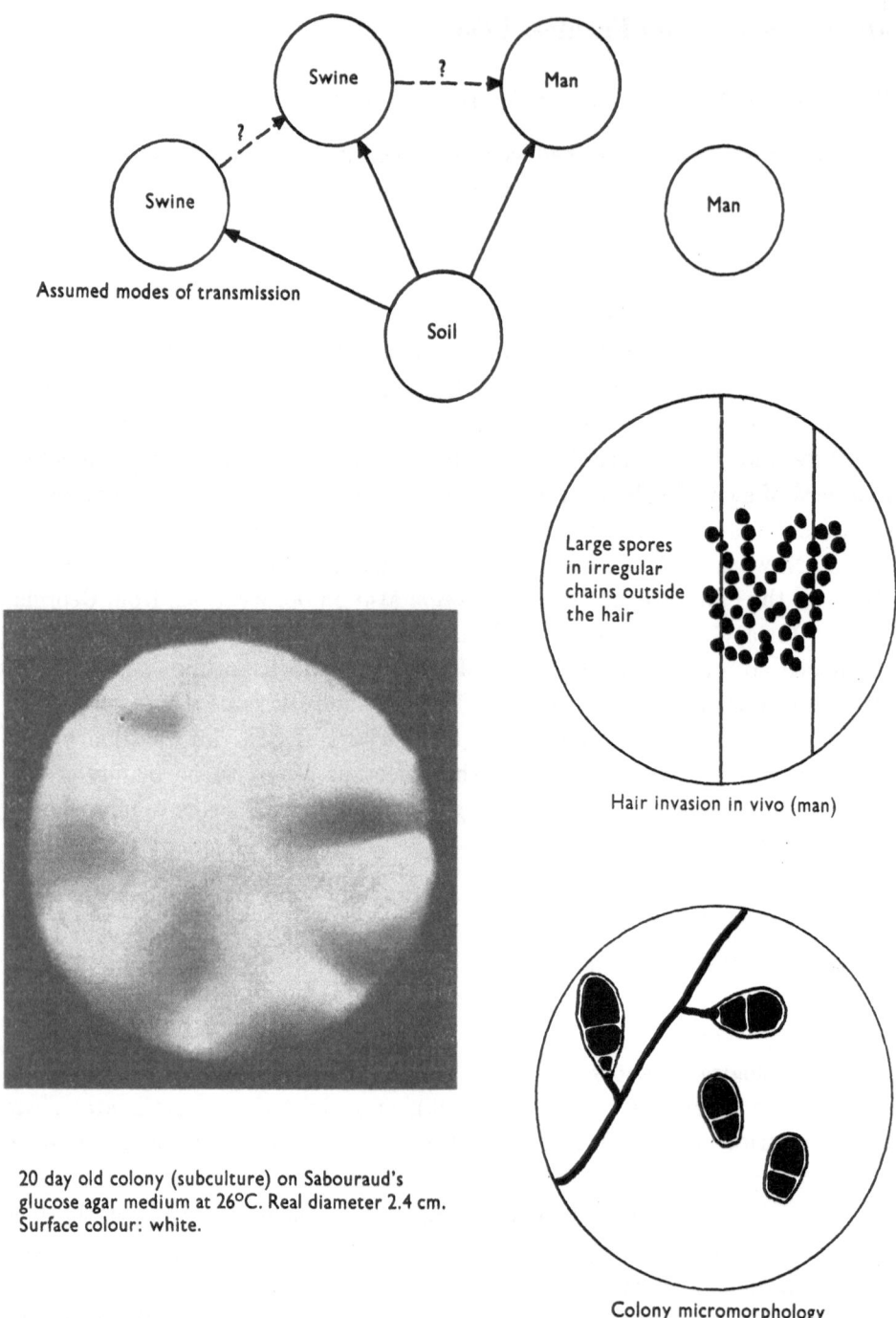

Assumed modes of transmission

Large spores in irregular chains outside the hair

Hair invasion in vivo (man)

20 day old colony (subculture) on Sabouraud's glucose agar medium at 26°C. Real diameter 2.4 cm. Surface colour: white.

Colony micromorphology

Fig. 34. *Microsporon nanum* Fuentes 1956. Dermatophyte occurring in soil, commonly attacking swine and occasionally infecting man.

reddened skin. Complications caused by acanthosis proliferating the skin have been reported by CARTER and GLENN (1966).

In man, tinea capitis and corporis have been observed. Hair invasion of the endoectothrix large spore type (5—8 μm). No fluorescence or very poor fluorescence of the infected hairs.

Direct microscopy

No hair invasion observed in pigs. In skin scrapings, pectinate highly branched septate hyphae (width 2·5 μm) are recorded. Human hair invasion reported to be of the endothrix or of the endoectothrix large spore type (5—8 μm).

Colony macromorphology

The colony attains a diameter of 20—35 mm after 10 days. The mature colony (after 10 days) has mostly a regular, circular to asteroid, but sometimes also an irregular asteroid ground plan. The surface can be powdery, velvety to fluffy flat or with some radial, shallow furrows. It can be white, gray, cream to cinnamon tan or salmon, pale lemon yellow to lemon yellow. At first, the surface can be saffron yellow, yellow or orange, later brownish red to dark red. Diffusible pigment is not produced.

Colony micromorphology

The most important diagnostic feature is the presence of abundant ovoid to pyriform, truncate, smooth or rough macroconidia with thin walls, 2—4 (mostly 2—3) cells, measuring 4—12 by 11—24 μm. Sometimes, macroconidia are not observed. Several strains produce ovoid, clavate to pyriform microconidia (1·5—2 by 4—5 μm), which are limited in numbers, sessile en thyrses (acladium type). Macroconidia sometimes are similar to those produced by *E. floccosum* or *K. ajelloi* var. *nana*.

Experimental pathogenicity

The culture is pathogenic for guinea-pigs and rabbits. No fluorescence of the hairs in the lesion.

Perfect state (*Nannizzia obtusa*):

Cleistothecium: size 250—450 μm.
Colour: buff.
Character of peridium: daughter hyphae form an obtuse angle with mother hyphae, curved towards the cleistothecium; verticillate branching is rare, cells with 1—2 constrictions.
Peridial appendages — tight spirals, tapered hyphae.

Trichophyton terrestre **Durie et Frey, 1957**

Perfect state: *Arthroderma lenticularum* Pore, Tsao et Plunkett, 1965, *Arthroderma quadrifidum* Dawson et Gentles, 1961.

Distribution

Terrestrial dermatophyte found in America, Asia, Australia and Europe, contaminating animals and man. Up to the present, however, no information is available on dermatophytoses caused by this fungus.

Colony macromorphology

The colony attains a diameter of 15—30 mm after 10 days. The mature colony (after 10 days) has mostly a regular ground plan — circular to asteroid. It is velvety to velvety powdered, flat. The surface colour is salmon, pale lemon yellow, pale yellow greenish, sometimes white at the periphery. The reverse can be saffron yellow, sienna, yellow or pale yellow greenish. No diffusible pigment produced.

Colony micromorphology

The most important diagnostic sign is the presence of numerous microconidia, macroconidia and transitional, intermediary forms of these spores. Microconidia are ovoid, clavate to pyriform, 2·5—5 by 3·5—6·5 μm. Macroconidia are cigar-shaped, smooth, with thin walls, 2—12 cells, 3—6 by 8—60 μm.

Experimental pathogenicity

Generally, the strains are completely apathogenic.

Keratinolysis of hairs in vitro

T. terrestre attacks rectangularly the hairs of man, coaxially the hairs of goat, horse and mouse and, in both ways, the hairs of cattle and dog.

Nutritional requirements
No special requirements.

Perfect state: (*Arthroderma lenticularum*):

Cleistothecium: size 300—600 μm.
Colour: light yellow.
Character of peridium: terminal branches of hyphae usually with more than three cells, cells dumbbell-shaped, strongly constricted, mostly symmetrical.
Peridial appendages — spirals of different length.

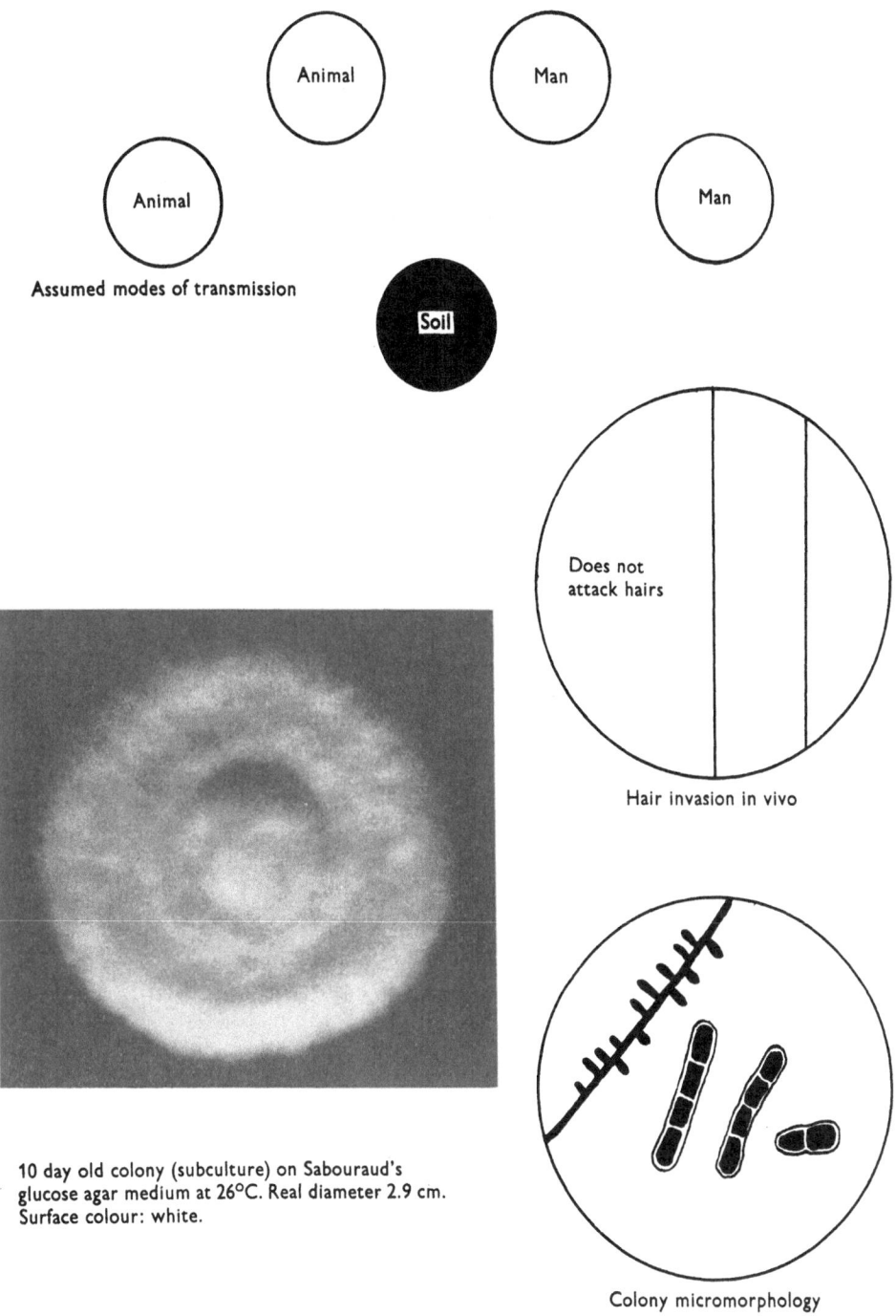

Animal

Man

Animal

Man

Assumed modes of transmission

Soil

Does not attack hairs

Hair invasion in vivo

10 day old colony (subculture) on Sabouraud's glucose agar medium at 26°C. Real diameter 2.9 cm. Surface colour: white.

Colony micromorphology

Fig. 35. *Trichophyton terrestre* Durie et Frey 1957. Apathogenic dermatophyte occurring in soil.

Perfect state: (*Arthroderma quadrifidum*)

Cleistothecium: size 400—700 μm.

Colour: light buff.

Character of peridium: cells of hyphae dumbbell-shaped, strongly constricted, asymmetrical. Their enlarged ends carry 1—2 protuberances on the external side of the hyphal turn.

Peridial appendages — spirals of different length.

Dermatophytes rarely isolated from animals and man

With the exception of *T. simii*, more or less typical subcultures of these dermatophytes could be studied in our laboratory. Until the present, these dermatophytes were not isolated in Czechoslovakia. *T. simii* was isolated from a monkey and described by PINOY (1912) as *E. simii*. There was no further evidence of this fungus until 1929, when Duncan obtained two isolates and deposited them in the culture collection of the London School of Hygiene and Tropical Medicine. In 1940, also Emmons isolated this fungus. In view of the scarcity of information on these dermatophytes, our data have been taken from an article by STOCKDALE, MACKENZIE and AUSTWICK (1965) and from Medical Mycology by DODGE (1937).

Microsporon distortum di Menna et Marples, 1954

Perfect state: not known.

Its identity with *M. umbonatum* Sabouraud, 1907 has been considered (FLÓRIÁN, GALGÓCZY and NOVÁK 1964).

Distribution

DI MENNA and MARPLES (1954) isolated 12 strains of this fungus from residents of New Zealand. KAPLAN et al. (1957) isolated it from 4 pet monkeys and one dog in the U.S.A., BROOKS, JOSEPH and CAMPBELL (1959) isolated it from a patient in the U.S.A., FREY, DURIE and BECKE (1960) from two children in Australia. Cat and monkey are suspected to be the source of human infection. BÜHLMAN and RIETH (1962) record the infection of guinea-pig and rabbit. In man, it causes tinea capitis (children) and tinea corporis (adults). Bright yellow-green fluorescence observed in invaded hairs of animal and man. Hair invasion of the endoectothrix small spore type (2—3 μm). Saprophytic habitat unknown.

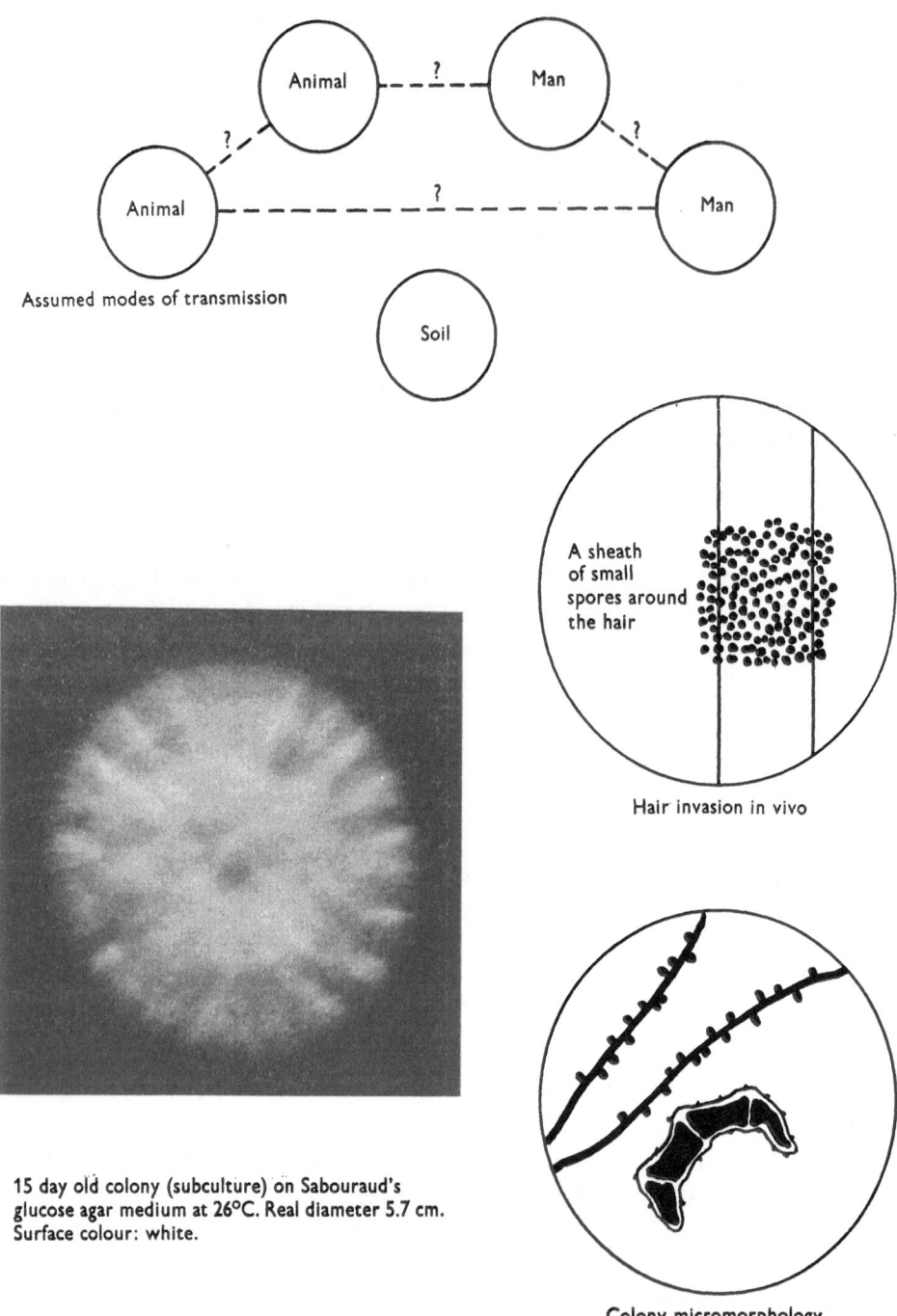

Assumed modes of transmission

A sheath
of small
spores around
the hair

Hair invasion in vivo

15 day old colony (subculture) on Sabouraud's
glucose agar medium at 26°C. Real diameter 5.7 cm.
Surface colour: white.

Colony micromorphology

Fig. 36. *Microsporon distortum* di Menna et Marples 1954. Infection of man and some animals, registered in North America and Australia.

Colony macromorphology

The colony attains a diameter of 30 mm after 14 days (the subculture of our strain obtained from Atlanta attained a diameter of 20—40 mm after 10 days). The mature colony (after 10 days) has mostly a regular ground plan — circular to asteroid. It is velvety fluffy; some radial shallow furrows may be present. Sometimes, the observed strains had little aerial mycelium and a waxy appearance. The surface colour varies from white, cream, tan to yellow brown in older cultures. The studied strain was completely white, salmon to pale lemon yellow or with a white margin. The reverse is colourless to dull yellowish tan or yellowish buff; in our strain it was salmon, apricot, pale lemon yellow to lemon yellow.

Colony micromorphology

The most important diagnostic feature is the presence of typical macroconidia, sometimes limited, sometimes abundant in occurrence. Their shape is irregular, contorted, resembling a sickle, rough, with thin walls, 3—10 cells, measuring 4 to 27 by 30—89 μm. Microconidia may be found in abundant or limited numbers, being clavate to pyriform in shape (1·5—4 by 3—11 μm) borne en thyrses (acladium type). Chandeliers, nodular bodies and spirals observed, chlamydospores are often formed.

Differential diagnosis

Sometimes, *M. distortum* must be differentiated from *M. audouinii*.

Experimental pathogenicity

Pathogenic for guinea-pigs.

Nutritional requirements

Nutritional requirements unknown.

Microsporon vanbreuseghemii Georg, Ajello, Friedman et Brinkman, 1962

Perfect state: *Nannizzia grubyia* Georg, Ajello, Friedman et Brinkman, 1962.

Distribution

GEORG et al. (1959) first isolated this fungus from a ringworm of a Malabar squirrel in Chicago Zoological Park. Later, it was isolated from a case of ring-

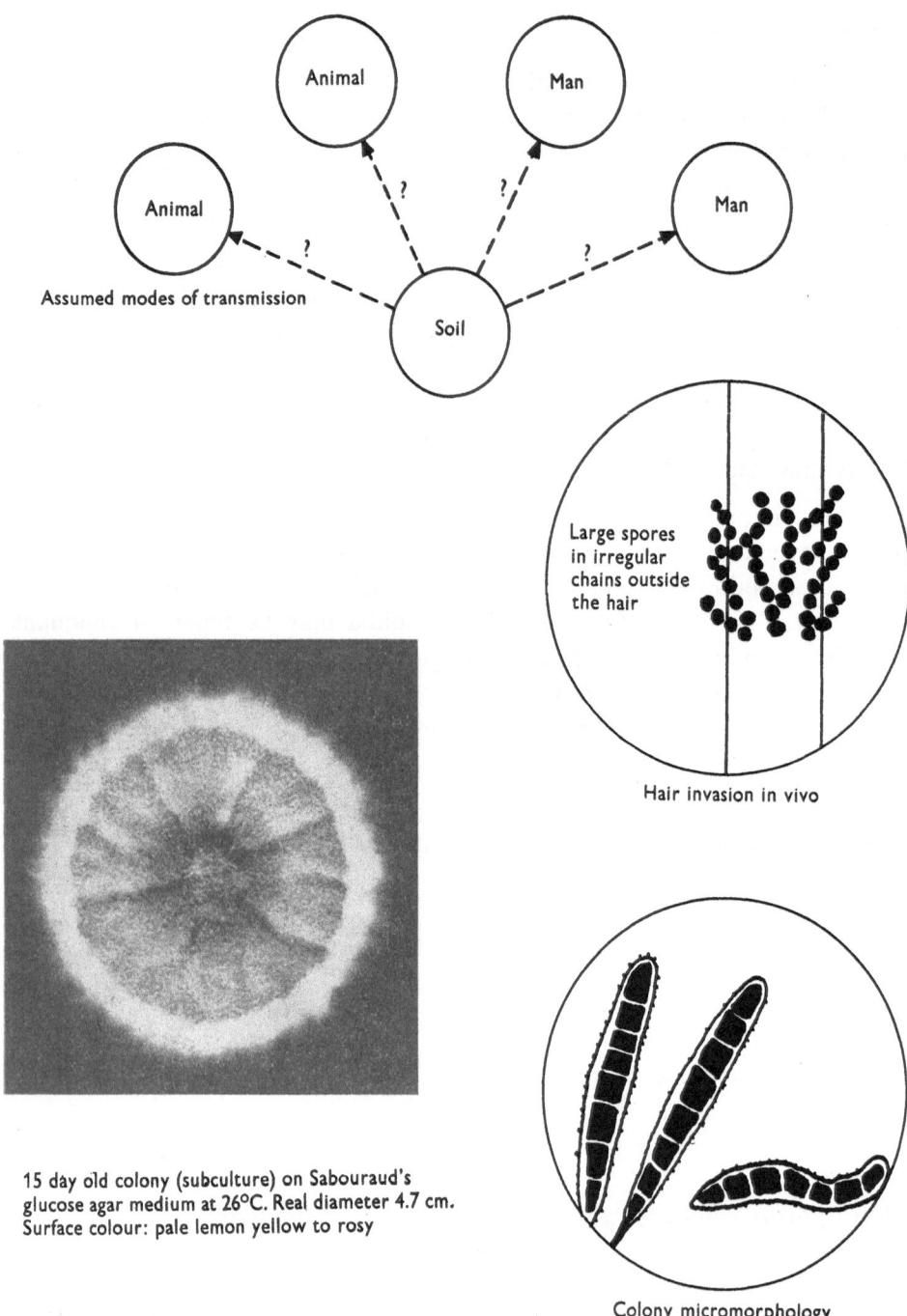

Animal

Man

Animal

Man

Assumed modes of transmission

Soil

Large spores
in irregular
chains outside
the hair

Hair invasion in vivo

15 day old colony (subculture) on Sabouraud's
glucose agar medium at 26°C. Real diameter 4.7 cm.
Surface colour: pale lemon yellow to rosy

Colony micromorphology

Fig. 37. *Microsporon vanbreuseghemii* Georg et al. 1962. Infection of man and some animals, registered in North America and Europe.

worm in a dog and in man. *M. vanbreuseghemii* has also been observed in Europe. In man, it causes tinea capitis. Hair invasion of the endoectothrix large spore type (5—8 μm). No or very poor fluorescence of infected hairs. Saprophytic habitat unknown, but infection may be of soil origin.

Colony macromorphology

The colony grows rapidly, attaining a diameter of 35—55 mm after 10 days. The mature colony (after 10 days) has mostly a regular ground plan — circular to asteroid. It is flat, granular to velvety, sometimes surrounded by a large zone of submerged mycelium. There is little tendency to wrinkle. The surface colour is white-yellowish or tan-pink-deep rose. The colour of our strain (subculture obtained from Atlanta) was completely pale rosy, pale lemon yellow to yellow or with a white margin. Pale lemon yellow to lemon yellow pigment diffusing into the environment of the colony. The reverse colour is light yellow to bright lemon yellow or orange, not pigmented, in our strain it was saffron yellow, orange, terra-cotta or yellow. "Pleomorphic degeneration" observable at an early stage.

Colony micromorphology

The most important diagnostic feature is the presence of abundant, spindle- to cigar-shaped, rough macroconidia with thick walls, 6—13 cells, measuring 8—13 by 44—88 μm. Microconidia usually numerous, ovoid, clavate to pyriform (3—6 by 4·5 to 13 μm), borne en thyrses (acladium type).

Experimental pathogenicity

Pathogenic for guinea-pigs. It must be differentiated especially from *K. ajelloi*.

Nutritional requirements

Nutritional requirements unknown.

Perfect state (*Nannizzia grubyia*):

Cleistothecium: size 150—600 μm.
Colour: light buff.
Character of peridium: hyphae curved towards cleistothecium, rarely branched in verticillate manner, cells of hyphae with a single constriction in the middle.
Peridial appendages — long spirals with up to 30—50 turns, tapered hyphae.

Trichophyton simii Pinoy, Stockdale, Mackenzie et Austwick, 1965

Perfect state: *Arthroderma simii* Stockdale, Mackenzie et Austwick, 1965.

Described in 1912 as *Epidermophyton simii*.

On the grounds of detailed studies of several strains, STOCKDALE, MACKENZIE and AUSTWICK (1965) re-established it as a species. Before that it was considered to belong to *T. mentagrophytes*.

Distribution

Attacks of chickens seem to be common, but isolations have also been recorded from monkey, man and dog, although in man only one case (tinea manus) has been satisfactorily described. Similar as other dermatophytes, for which a perfect state has been found, this dermatophyte may also saprophytize in soil. Until the present, all anamnestically clear cases originated in India.

Colony macromorphology

The colony generally covers the petri dish (84 mm) after two weeks and is velvety with a finely granular surface and a fluffy, asteroid margin. The surface is pale buff, the reverse straw- to salmon-coloured.

Colony micromorphology

The most important diagnostic sign is the presence of numerous cigar- to spindle-shaped, smooth macroconidia with thin walls, 5—11 cells. In young colonies, microconidia are rare, but more abundant in old ones. They are clavate to pyriform (1·5—3 by 2—6·5 μm), borne en thyrses (acladium type). Spirals are present.

Differential diagnosis

T. simii must be differentiated from *T. mentagrophytes*.

Experimental pathogenicity

Pathogenic for guinea-pigs; hair invasion of the endoectothrix large spore type.

Nutritional requirements

No requirements for thiamine or inositol.

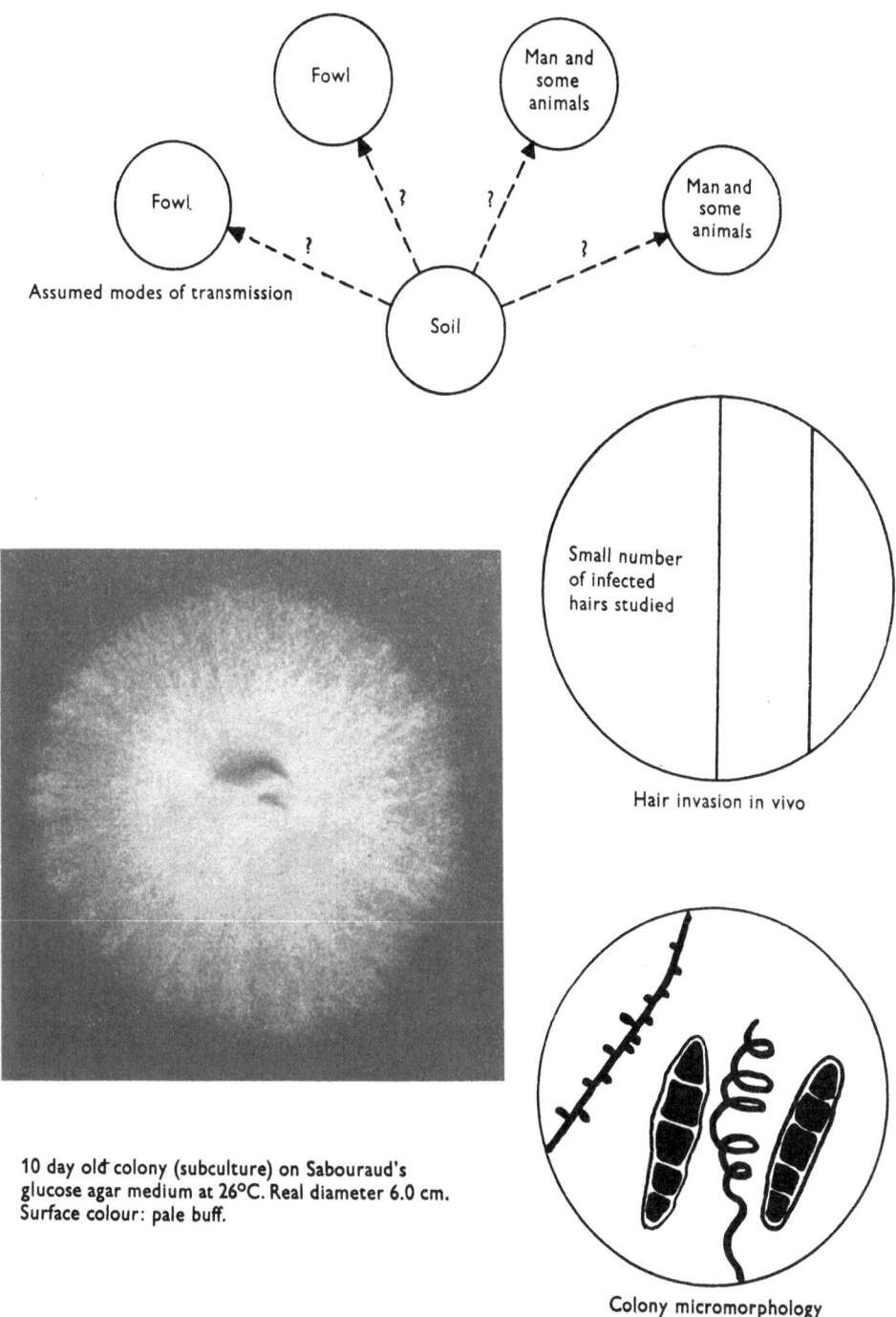

Fowl

Man and some animals

Fowl

Man and some animals

Assumed modes of transmission

?

?

?

?

Soil

Small number of infected hairs studied

Hair invasion in vivo

10 day old colony (subculture) on Sabouraud's glucose agar medium at 26°C. Real diameter 6.0 cm. Surface colour: pale buff.

Colony micromorphology

Fig. 38. *Trichophyton simii* Pinoy et al. 1965. Infection of animals (especially fowl) and man, registered in India.

Perfect state (*Arthroderma simii*):

Cleistothecium: size 200—750 μm.

Colour: light buff.

Character of peridium: terminal branches of hyphae with 2—3 cells at the utmost, sometimes verticillate branching of hyphae, cells of internal peridial hyphae clavate, of outer hyphae dumbbell-shaped, strongly constricted, mostly symmetrical.

Peridial appendages — long spirals with up to 20—30 turns.

Anthropophilic dermatophytes which do not attack animals

These dermatophytes are not endemic in Czechoslovakia. Only the species *M. ferrugineum* has been isolated here, which was mostly in connection with Korean children, brought to live in Czechoslovakia (LANGER 1953, MANYCH and KEJDA 1966). HEJTMÁNEK (1957) published an interesting comparative study of six strains of *M. ferrugineum*. All descriptions of anthropophilic dermatophytes which do not attack animals were taken from the literature and from the results of our studies of numerous strains obtained from various laboratories.

Microsporon ferrugineum Ota, 1922

Perfect state: not known.

Some authors have placed it to *Trichophyta*. Recently, GEORG et al. (1963) and VARSAVSKY and AJELLO (1964) retransferred it to Microspora.

Distribution

Saprophytic source unknown. Probably only interhuman propagation, animal dermatophytoses not registered. Human infection common in some parts of Africa, Asia and Europe. Reported mainly as the cause of tinea capitis in children. Less frequent is tinea corporis, rare tinea barbae and unguium. Hair invasion of the endoectothrix small spore type (2—3 μm). Bright yellow fluorescence of infected hairs.

Colony macromorphology

The colony attains a diameter of 10—30 mm after 10 days. The mature colony (after 15 days) may have a regular, circular to asteroid, or irregularly asteroid, polygonal to lobulate ground plan. It is either entirely glabrous or membranous with some granulations or filaments, sometimes velvety or granular. Some

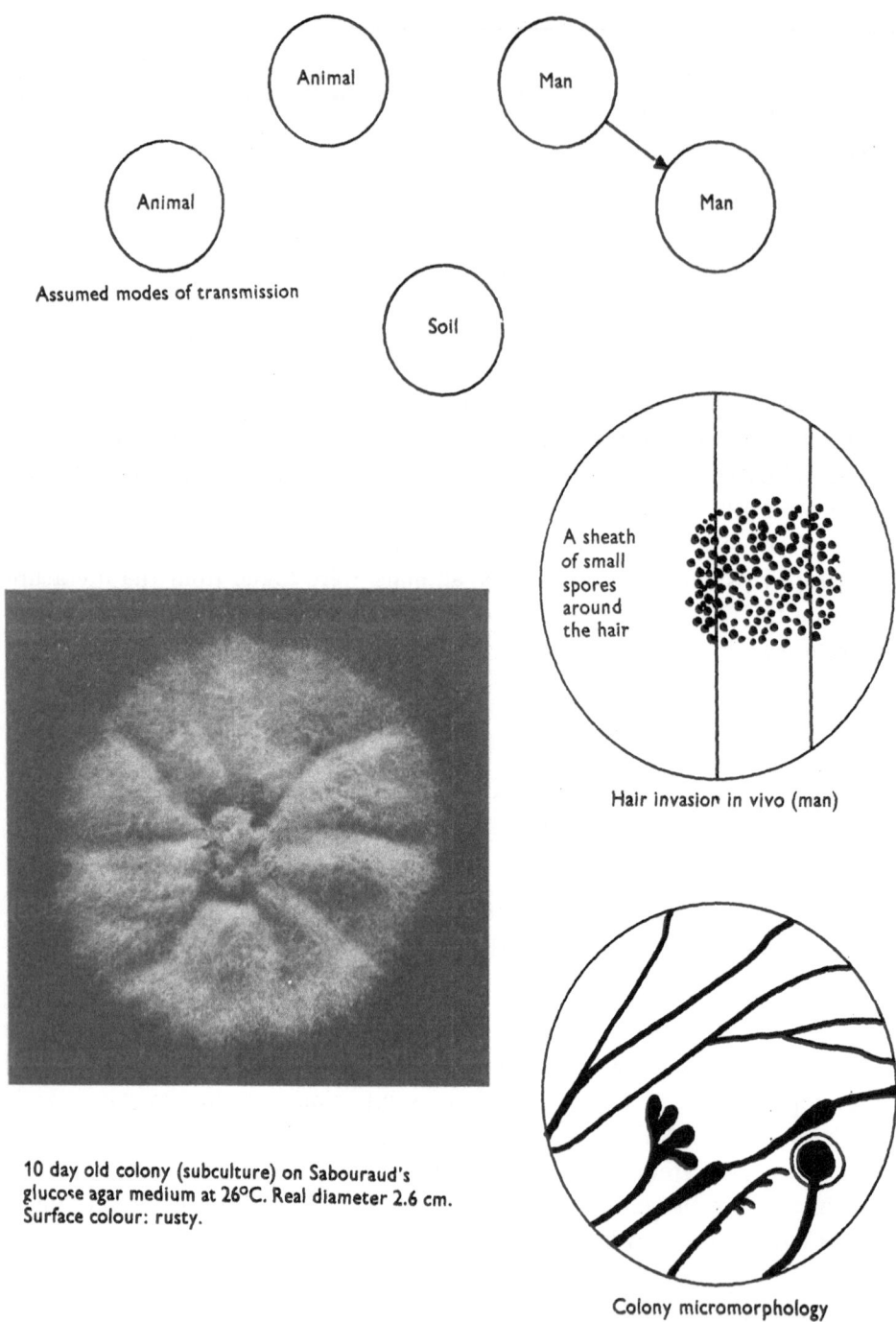

Animal

Animal

Assumed modes of transmission

Man

Man

Soil

A sheath
of small
spores
around
the hair

Hair invasion in vivo (man)

10 day old colony (subculture) on Sabouraud's
glucose agar medium at 26°C. Real diameter 2.6 cm.
Surface colour: rusty.

Colony micromorphology

Fig. 39. *Microsporon ferrugineum* (Ota) Langeron et Milochevitch 1930. Infection
of man, registered in Africa, Asia and Europe.

strains produce abundant submerged mycelium, whereby the aerial part of the colony remains underdeveloped. The colonies show a marked tendency to wrinkle, to form furrows and folds. Fissures appear in older colonies. The surface may be of various colour, but mostly, the strains are yellowish to deep rust. They can also be rosy, red, blood red, carmine, salmon, apricot, saffron yellow, rusty terra-cotta, pale lemon yellow, lemon yellow, yellow or yellow greenish. The reverse is usually dull orange, but may also be blood red, carmine, dark blood red, saffron yellow to yellow or without pigment. Some authors separate *M. ferrugineum* var. *album*, being flatter and with a white, downy surface.

Colony micromorphology

The micromorphology is poor. Macroconidia and microconidia are not produced. Exceptionally, the swollen endings of the hyphae, resembling macroconidia and pyriform microconidia are found. Favic chandeliers, pectinate hyphae, racquets may be present. Chlamydospores are usually numerous.

Differential diagnosis

Sometimes, it must be differentiated from *T. sudanense*.

Experimental pathogenicity

Pathogenicity for laboratory animals is low. Most of the tested strains were completely incapable of producing lesions on guinea-pigs.

Nutritional requirements

No special requirements.

Trichophyton concentricum Blanchard, 1896

Perfect state: not known.

Distribution

Saprophytic source unknown. Probably only interhuman propagation, animal dermatophytoses not registered. Infection of man common in the Pacific Islands. Also reported from Central and South America and Asia. Causes a special dermatophytosis (tinea corporis) named tinea imbricata or tokelau. Occasionally, nails are invaded, hairs are not attacked.

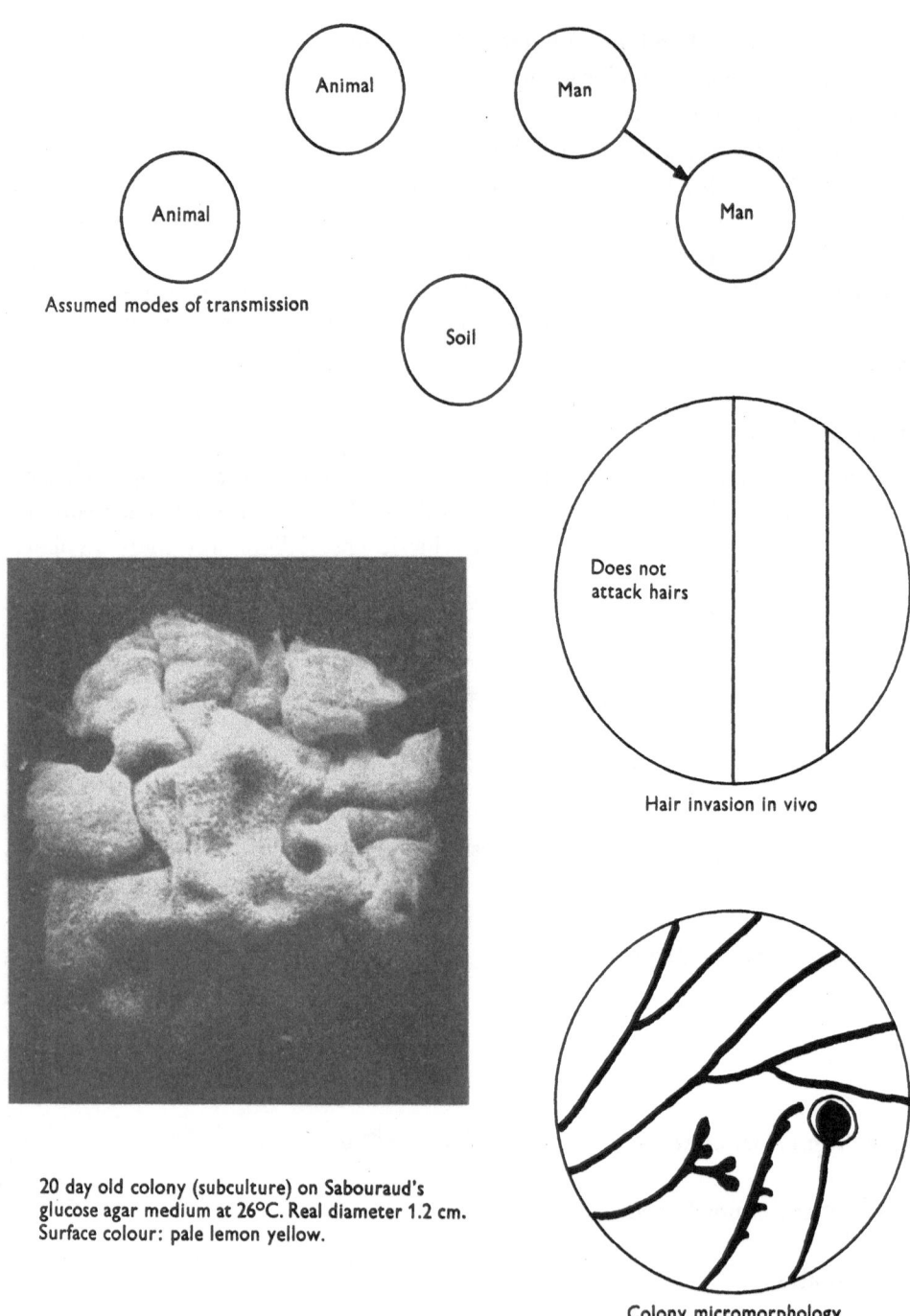

Animal

Animal

Man

Man

Assumed modes of transmission

Soil

Does not
attack hairs

Hair invasion in vivo

20 day old colony (subculture) on Sabouraud's
glucose agar medium at 26°C. Real diameter 1.2 cm.
Surface colour: pale lemon yellow.

Colony micromorphology

Fig. 40. *Trichophyton concentricum* Blanchard 1896. Infection of man, registered
mainly in Oceania.

Colony macromorphology

The colony attains a diameter of 5—20 mm after 10 days. The mature colony (after 20 days) may have a regular — circular to asteroid, or irregularly polygonal to lobulate ground plan. It is glabrous, more often membranous, slightly powdered to velvety. The colonies are raised, there is a marked tendency to wrinkle, to form furrows and folds. Fissures may appear in older colonies. The surface colour varies. In some strains the surface is almost uniformly coloured, but sometimes, the margin and centre are of different colour or there are differently coloured patches. Mostly, the strains are white to grayish, changing into cream and amber. The following colours were observed on the surface: white to gray, vinaceous, reddish, salmon, apricot, saffron yellow, orange, pale lemon yellow. The reverse is terra-cotta or pale lemon yellow. Sometimes, diffusible pigment coloured lemon yellow to yellow has been observed.

Colony micromorphology

The micromorphology is poor. Macroconidia and microconidia are not produced. Favic chandeliers and pectinate hyphae are occasionally present. Chlamydospores are generally numerous.

Differential diagnosis

It must sometimes be differentiated from *T. schoenleinii* or *T. verrucosum*.

Experimental pathogenicity

Pathogenicity for laboratory animals is low. Most of the tested strains were completely incapable of producing lesions.

Nutritional requirements

No special requirements. About 50% of the strains studied were stimulated by thiamine and by certain thiazole compounds.

Trichophyton gourvilii Catanei, 1933

Some authors considered it to be in synonymy with *T. violaceum*. Recently e.g. VARSAVSKY and AJELLO (1964) recommended its separation as a valid species.

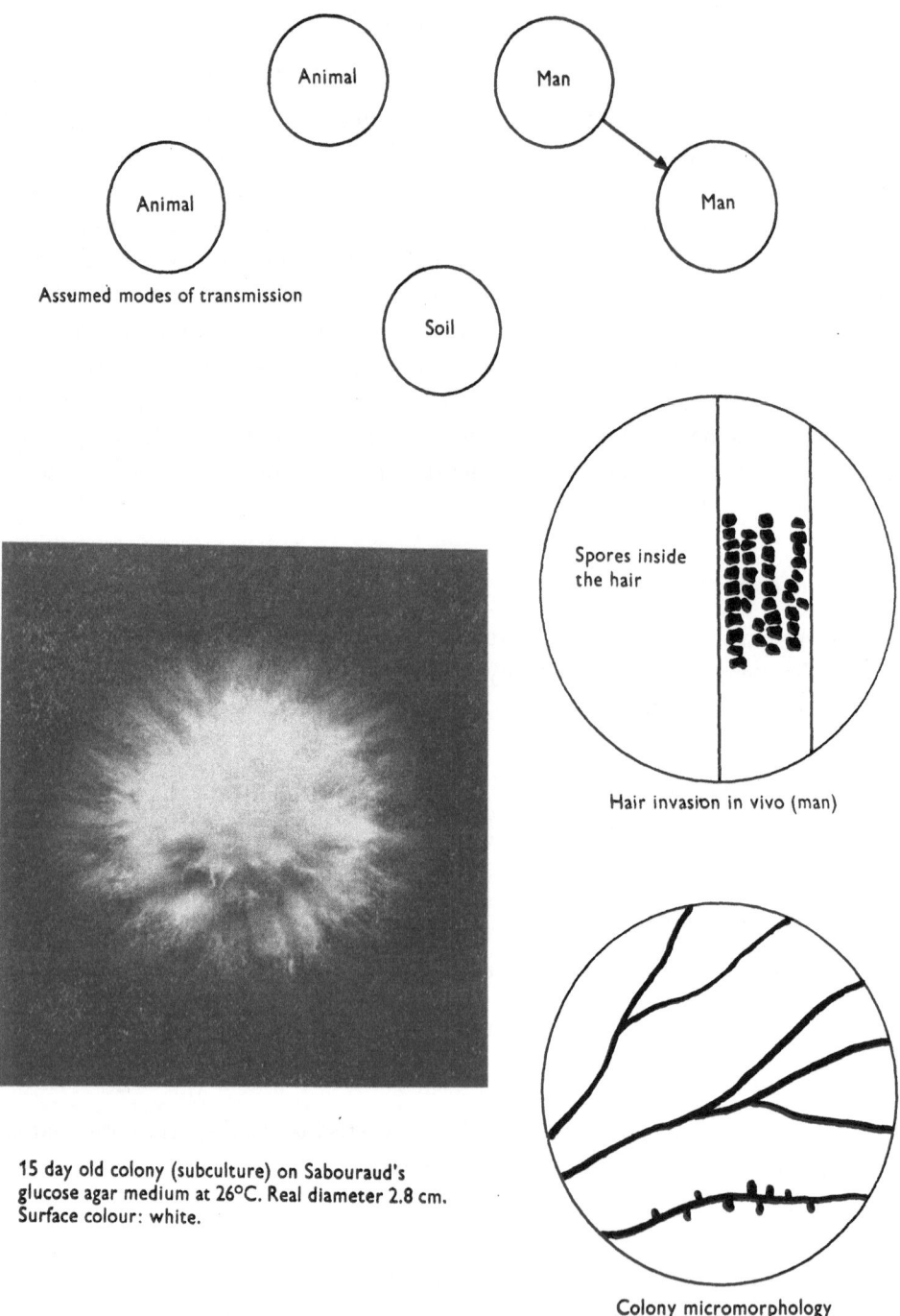

Assumed modes of transmission

Spores inside the hair

Hair invasion in vivo (man)

15 day old colony (subculture) on Sabouraud's glucose agar medium at 26°C. Real diameter 2.8 cm. Surface colour: white.

Colony micromorphology

Fig. 41. *Trichophyton gourvilii* Catanei 1933. Infection of man, registered in Africa.

Distribution

Saprophytic source unknown. Probably only interhuman propagation, animal dermatophytoses not registered. Human infection common in some parts of Africa. Reported as the cause of tinea capitis and corporis. Hair invasion of the endothrix type. The colony attains a diameter of 10—30 mm after 10 days. The mature colony (after 15 days) may have a regular — circular to asteroid — or irregularly asteroid ground plan. It is membranous, glabrous and waxy, later shortly velvety, more or less wrinkled or folded. The surface is white, gray lavender, violet to deep garnet red. The reverse is salmon, pale lemon yellow. Macroconidia mostly not found, in some strains present in limited numbers. They are of irregular shape, smooth, with thin walls, 5—9 cells, measuring 4—8 by 25—45 μm. In some strains microconidia not observed, in others present in limited numbers. They are ovoid, clavate to pyriform, 1—4 by 2—5 μm.

Differential diagnosis

Sometimes it must be differentiated from *T. violaceum*.

Experimental pathogenicity

Pathogenic for guinea-pigs.

Nutritional requirements

Nutritional requirements not known.

Trichophyton sudanense Joyeux, 1912

Perfect state: not known.

Distribution

Saprophytic source unknown. Probably only interhuman propagation, animal dermatophytoses not registered. Several cases, probably of African origin, recently reported from Europe by HAUSER and HEYMER (1964), KABEN (1964), SCHÖNBORN (1966) and from America by RIPPON and MEDENICA (1964). Mainly recorded as the cause of tinea capitis and corporis, sporadically also of tinea pedis and unguium.

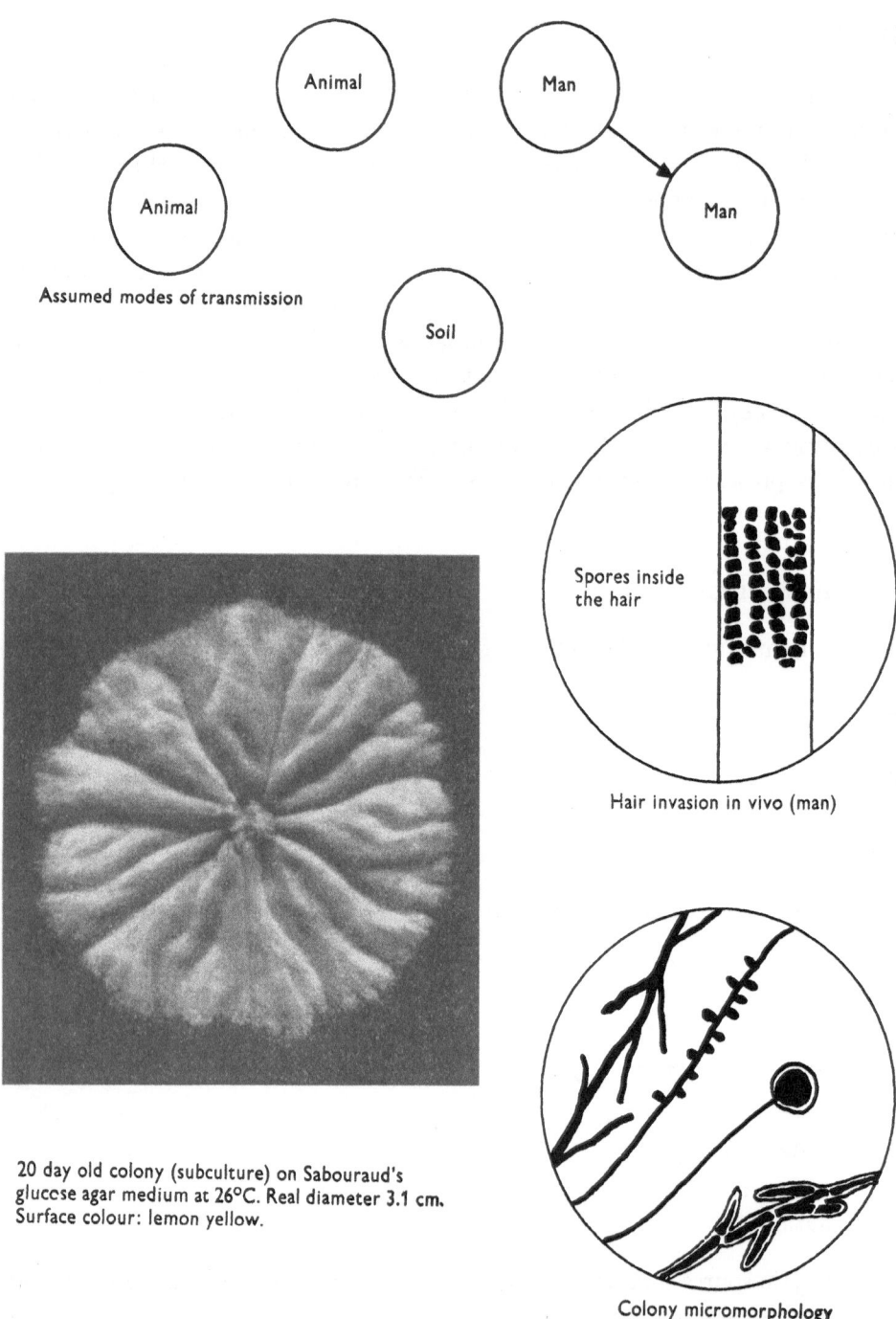

Animal

Man

Animal

Man

Assumed modes of transmission

Soil

Spores inside the hair

Hair invasion in vivo (man)

20 day old colony (subculture) on Sabouraud's glucose agar medium at 26°C. Real diameter 3.1 cm. Surface colour: lemon yellow.

Colony micromorphology

Fig. 42. *Trichophyton sudanense* Joyeux 1912. Infection of man, registered in Africa.

Colony macromorphology

The colony attains a diameter of 5—20 mm after 10 days. The mature colony (after 15 days) may have a regular – circular to asteroid – or irregularly asteroid to lobulate ground plan. It is membranous powdery to velvety with a relatively dense aerial mycelium. The colonies, at first flat, become raised, showing a marked tendency to wrinkle, to form furrows and folds. The surface may be variously coloured, white, yellow to orange, lemon yellow (often the colour of a dried apricot). The reverse can be saffron yellow, yellow to orange, yellow to brown.

Colony micromorphology

This species is know by its special type of hyphal branching. Macroconidia are not produced. Microconidia are few or numerous, mostly present in limited numbers, ovoid, clavate to pyriform (2—3 by 3—7 µm), developing mainly from the sides of the hyphae (acladium type), but even en grappes (botrytis type). Chlamydospores can be abundant especially in older cultures.

Differential diagnosis

T. sudanense must sometimes be differentiated from *M. ferrugineum*.

Experimental pathogenicity

Pathogenicity for laboratory animals is low. The tested strains were incapable of producing lesions.

Nutritional requirements

No special requirements.

*Trichophyton yaoundei** Cochet, Doby-Dubois, Deblock et Vaiva, 1957

Perfect state: not known.

GEORG et al. (1963) proved in a detailed study the validity of *T. yaoundei* as a species.

Distribution

Saprophytic source unknown. Probably only interhuman propagation, animal dermatophytoses not registered. Human infection common in some parts

* An area of the Cameroon known as Yaoundé.

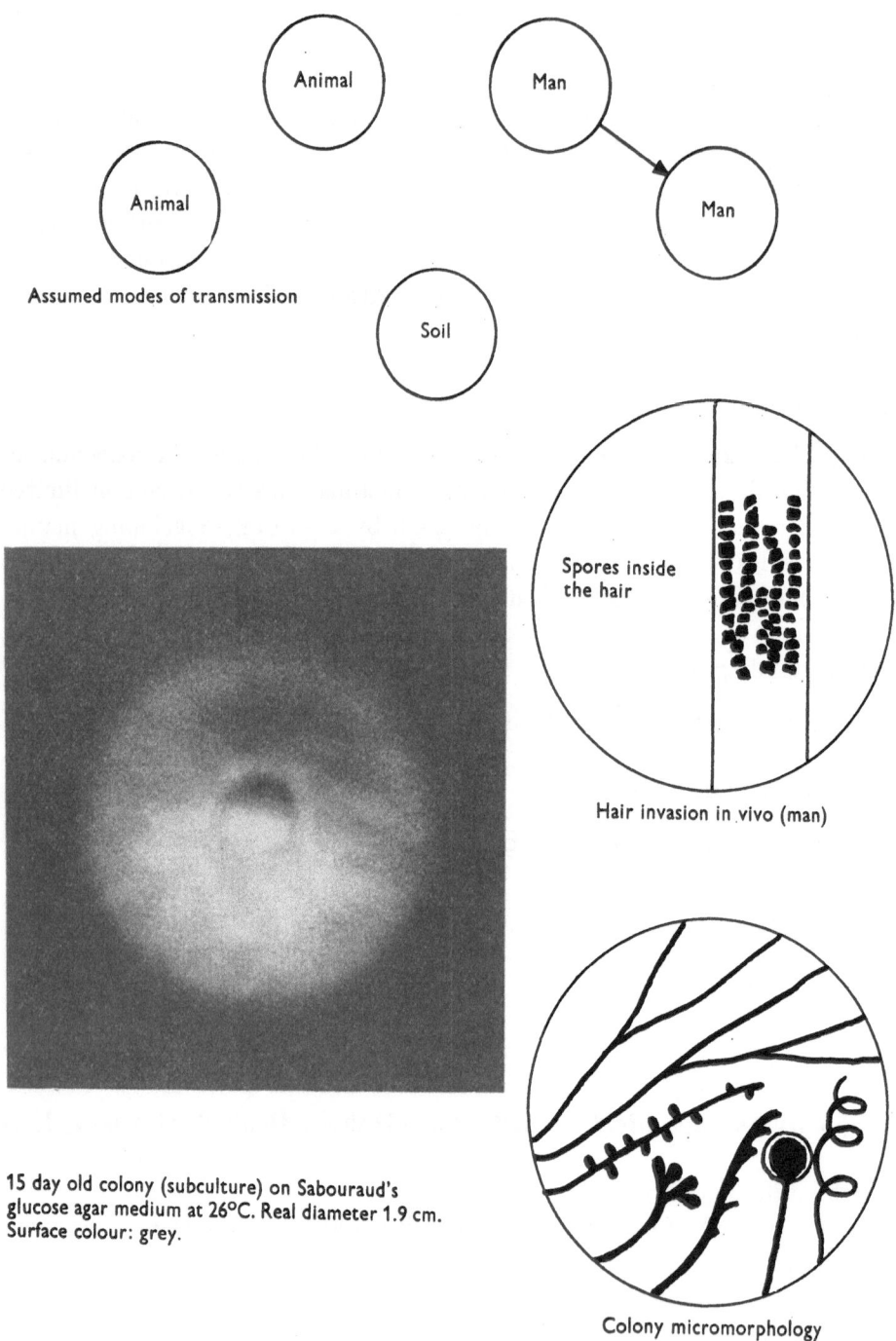

Assumed modes of transmission

Spores inside the hair

Hair invasion in vivo (man)

15 day old colony (subculture) on Sabouraud's glucose agar medium at 26°C. Real diameter 1.9 cm. Surface colour: grey.

Colony micromorphology

Fig. 43. *Trichophyton yaoundei* Cochet et al. 1957. Infection of man, registered in Africa.

of Africa. SARKANY and MIDGLEY (1966) isolated it in England from two negro children from the West Cameroon. Reported as the cause of tinea capitis. Hair invasion of the endothrix type.

Colony macromorphology

The colony attains a diameter of 5—20 mm after 10 days. The mature colony (after 20 days) may have a regular — circular to asteroid — or irregularly asteroid, polygonal to lobulate ground plan. It is glabrous, more often membranous, sometimes slightly powdered to short velvety. The colonies are raised, showing a tendency to form furrows and folds. Some strains grow submerged in the agar. The surface may be white, yellow, cream, in older colonies tan to brown. The reverse is unpigmented or, in older colonies, brown. Sometimes, this brown pigment diffuses into the environment of the colony.

Subcultures grow more rapidly than primary isolates, their colour may be darker.

Colony micromorphology

Macroconidia are not produced. Microconidia are absent or present in limited numbers — they are ovoid, clavate to pyriform (1 by 1·5—2·5 µm), produced along the sides of the simple hyphae (acladium type). Some strains produce them on casein agar. Favic chandeliers may be numerous, pectinate hyphae and spirals occasionally found. Chlamydospores, especially in older cultures, may be abundant.

Differential diagnosis

T. yaoundei must sometimes be differentiated from *T. verrucosum* and *T. violaceum*.

Experimental pathogenicity

Apathogenic for guinea-pigs.

Nutritional requirements

No special requirements.

Dermatophytes of doubtful systematic position

With the exception of *Sabouraudites praecox*, none of the dermatophytes could be studied in our laboratory. However, even *S. praecox* will soon become irreversibly atypical. Findings of *M. equinum*, *S. langeronii*, *T. persicolor* and *T. sulphureum* have repeatedly been reported.

Microsporon equinum Bodin, 1896

Considered in synonymy with *M. canis*, a conception not accepted by some mycologists (e.g. AUSTWICK 1966). Should not be mistaken for *T. equinum!* Causes equine ringworm transmissible to man.

The colony is membranous, radially furrowed, producing diffusible yellow pigment. Pyriform microconidia en grappes, numerous macroconidia, echinulated, measuring 18—20 by 25—35 µm. Pathogenic for guinea-pigs; hair invasion of the endoectothrix type.

Sabouraudites duboisii Vanbreuseghem, 1949

Isolated from a European child in the ex-Belgian Congo (VANBREUSEGHEM 1949).

The colony grows rapidly and is circular to asteroid. The centre is velvety and white, the periphery powdered and orange. The reverse is yellowish. Macroconidia numerous, cylindrical, pointed, rough, with thin walls, mostly 6 cells, measuring 8—9 by 50—60 µm. Numerous pyriform microconidia (1·5—2 by 5—6 µm). Pathogenic for the guinea-pig; hair invasion of the endo-ectothrix type.

Sabouraudites langeronii Vanbreuseghem, 1950

Repeatedly isolated in Africa (ex-Belgian Congo, Ruanda Urundi) from tinea capitis in children (VANBREUSEGHEM 1950).

Similar as *M. audouinii*, its distinct value as a species is disputable. Endoectothrix hair invasion of the small spore type. The colony attains a diameter of 10 mm after 7 days. It is circular to asteroid, velvety salmon to rosy coloured. The reverse is rosy. Pyriform microconidia and irregular macroconidia produced in limited numbers. Pathogenic for the guinea-pig.

Sabouraudites praecox Rivalier, 1954

In France, isolated from tinea corporis of a man (RIVALIER 1954).

The colony grows rapidly, its ground plan is circular; it is powdered to granular and yellowish-brownish in the centre with a velvety, white periphery. The surface is entirely flat. The reverse is orange. Numerous cigar-shaped, smooth macroconidia with thin walls, 2—9 cells, measuring 9—10 by 30—76 μm, are present.

Trichophyton persicolor Sabouraud, 1910

Considered as a synonym of *T. mentagrophytes*, a conception not accepted by some prominent mycologists. Although ringworm of a dog has been reported (AUSTWICK 1966), it seems to be anthropophilic.

The colony is circular, flat, powdered, rose coloured. Numerous microconidia are sometimes observed. Spirals present. Pathogenicity for guinea-pigs low.

Trichophyton rodhainii Vanbreuseghem, 1949

Isolated from tinea cruris (VANBREUSEGHEM 1949).

The colony grows slowly. It is membranous, raised and wrinkled, deep violet, later covered with white velvet. Microconidia are spherical to pyriform, macroconidia rare (3—4 cells, 5 by 30 μm). Pathogenic for the guinea-pig; hair invasion of the endothrix large spore type.

Trichophyton sulphureum Fox, 1908

Considered in synonymy with or as a variety of *T. tonsurans*. Sometimes referred to as a species (e.g. BEARE 1958). Known as the cause of tinea capitis and corporis.

At first, the colony is velvety and white, later orange powdered with a red centre and yellowish periphery. Some strains produce diffusible yellow pigment. Microconidia numerous, produced both en thyrses and en grappes. Macroconidia rare. Pathogenicity for the guinea-pig low, some strains are apathogenic.

Newly described dermatophytes

Except *T. vanbreuseghemii*, none of these dermatophytes could be studied in our laboratory up to the present. However, after several passages, also the mentioned *T. vanbreuseghemii* differed considerably from the original description of the culture. We are, therefore, giving only a brief description of these dermatophytes.

Keratinomyces longifusus Flórián et Galgóczy, 1964

Isolated in Hungary from tinea capitis and soil (FLÓRIÁN and GALGÓCZY 1964).

Perfect state: not known.

The colony grows rapidly, attaining a diameter of about 45 mm after 14 days. It is circular, velvety powdered, flat with a central umbo. The surface is white, pale yellowish, the reverse yellowish-brown. The most important diagnostic sign is the presence of numerous clavate, smooth macroconidia with thin walls, 4—15 cells, measuring 7—9 by 35—300 µm. Microconidia are not produced. Nodular bodies, racquets and chlamydospores may occur. The culture has been found to be apathogenic.

Microsporon rivalierii Vanbreuseghem, 1963

Isolated and described under the name *Sabouraudites rivalierii* from tinea capitis in Leopoldville. A valid Latin description given later by VANBREUSEG-HEM (1963). Several cases reported from Leopoldville.

Perfect state: not known.

The colony is snow white, very slightly downy. The centre is moderately depressed and 3—4 radial grooves are found on the surface. The reverse is light yellow tan. A few spindle-shaped, echinulate macroconidia of 6—7 cells, measuring 16—18 by 80—100 μm, are observed; often, their central diameter is smaller. Vegetative hyphae grow and branch, forming arches. No information available on its pathogenicity. Human hair invasion of the endoectothrix small spore type.

Thallomicrosporon kuehnii Benedek, 1963

One strain isolated from tinea capitis in the U.S.A. (BENEDEK 1964).

Perfect state: not known.

The colony grows very rapidly, attaining a diameter of about 70 mm after 10 days. It is woolly-velvety, white. The reverse is light yellow. The most important diagnostic sign is the presence of numerous macroconidia, formed directly in the vegetative mycelium (thallus). No sporophores bearing macroconidia are found. The macroconidia (the macroconidia-like thallospores) are spindle-shaped elements, with thin walls, 3—7 cells measuring 4—8 by 14 to 53 μm. The microconidia are rod-shaped to pyriform. Arthrospores forming rectangles, and rare chlamydospores are produced. No data available on its pathogenicity.

Trichophyton georgii Varsavsky et Ajello, 1964

Isolated from soil and the hairs of the opossum in the U.S.A. (VARSAVSKY and AJELLO 1964).

Perfect state: *Arthroderma ciferrii* Varsavsky et Ajello, 1964.

The centre of the colony is downy, pale grayish vinaceous. The flat area surrounding the umbonate centre is finely powdered to granular, indian lake to vinaceous brown. Periphery granular to floccose, pale brownish vinaceous, with irregularly fringed edges. The reverse of the colony is diamine brown, irregularly spotted with dark Indian red or dark vinaceous brown. Macroconidia not produced. Microconidia abundant, generally elongate clavate, sporadically pyriform or subglobose. Although generally nonseptate, 2—3 septations are sometimes present. Microconidia of a single cell measure 2—2·4 by 4·2—6·4 μm. The culture was found apathogenic.

Trichophyton vanbreuseghemii Rioux, Jarry et Juminer, 1964

Isolated from soil in Tunisia (RIOUX, JARRY and JUMINER 1964).

Perfect state: not known.

The colony attains a diameter of 30 mm after 5 days. It is velvety to powdery, whitish to yellowish, flat or radially folded. The reverse is yellowish-brownish. Numerous cylindrical or clavate macroconidia with thin walls, 5—8 cells, measuring 7—8 by 35 — 44 µm, are produced. Also pyriform microconidia (2—2·5 by 4—6 µm) are present. Abundant spirals were observed. The culture was found to be apathogenic.

No data concerning *Microsporon racemosum* Borelli, 1965 and *Trichophyton lipoferum* Kominami, 1960 have been available to us up to the present.

C. TECHNIQUES

I. EQUIPMENT FOR SAMPLE COLLECTION

The choice of instruments for collecting samples from dermatophytic lesions of animals depends on their character. Mostly the hairy parts of the skin are affected and the epidermal scales have to be scraped off together with the hairs. The basic instruments are scalpels, cyretes and epilating or anatomical tweezers. The hairs must be removed with their intrafollicular parts, therefore clipping is not satisfactory. Scissors are only used for cutting hair around inaccessible minute lesions.

Furthermore, sterile instruments should be used in field work and it is advisable to have a set in store. The same instrument should never be used twice for collecting samples from lesions of different specimens or different animal species even if the animals were kept in the same place. In very urgent cases the lack of suitable instruments can be overcome by sterilizing used scalpels or tweezers over the flame of a burner. Bacteriological wire loops are used for taking pus or serous exudate from pustular or vesicular efflorescences. Cotton wool tampons are used only exceptionally, when the lesions are not accessible in any other way (e.g. the auditory passage).

Samples are kept in sterile, wide-mouthed tubes with cork stoppers or in petri dishes. Rubber stoppered tubes are not suitable because of retaining a high relative humidity in the environment, enabling spore germination of contaminating saprophytes. The containers with the samples must be labelled (date of collection, animal species and address of sender — the attending veterinarian). Should not enough glass be available, the material may be kept between two sterile slides, wrapped in sterile paper.

Foci of animal dermatophytoses being always soiled must be cleaned immediately before collecting the specimens. A mixture of alcohol and benzine in equal parts or 96% alcohol, in which a swab of sterile cotton-wool, a gauze sponge or a cotton-wool tampon has been soaked, is suitable for decontamination.

When using Mackenzie's collecting technique, the fur of the animal must be combed with sterile brushes or metal combs. A sterile tooth-brush can be used for small animals.

II. COLLECTING MATERIAL FOR EXAMINATION

Reliable examination results can be obtained only by strictly observing all principles of specimen collection. Any deviation from these principles can unfavourably influence further work with the samples and lead to erroneous diagnostic conclusions.

The mode of collection depends on two factors: whether the disease is clinically apparent, i.e. with distinct, characteristic lesions or, whether a latent infection without apparent pathological changes is assumed.

In the first case we are searching the animal for fresh signs of the disease; after sterilizing the affected area, hairs, epidermal scales and larger parts of the defoliating skin are collected with suitable instruments and transferred into sterile containers. Mostly, the fur of the animals is considerably contaminated by saprophytic organisms, in particular with rapidly growing ubiquitous moulds, which are most undesirable for further work with the samples. Therefore, primary decontamination procedures are of such utmost importance.

The character of dermatophytic lesions of animals belonging to the same species is partly determined by the species, to which the pathological agent belongs, by the location of the lesion and by the age of the pathological process. The location of the lesion is influenced not only by the affinity of the dermatophyte, but often also by predisposing factors; of these, the most distinct is the dependence on sites exposed to trauma and microtrauma. The most affected parts are the head, the neck and the extremities. Only in subsequent stages of the infection are lesions formed on other parts of the body. Specimens should be collected from more than one lesion on the same animal and, whenever possible, from different parts of the body. In clearly identical infection of the whole herd, the same breed etc., the examination of only 3—5 animals with typical and fresh signs of the disease is sometimes sufficient.

Dry, noninflammatory or only slightly inflamed foci with fallen out or broken off hairs are easily decontaminated and epidermal scales can be collected with a scalpel or a cyrete. Also parasitized hairs can be collected with little difficulty. Special attention should be paid to hairs altered by the infection (discoloured hairs broken off close to the surface of the epidermis etc.). The collection of specimens from infiltrated areas or from areas affected by heavy exudative secretion is more difficult. The examiner often finds small crusts or a crusty layer and bunches of hairs stuck together with exudate. The secretion of the exudate is particularly distinct on an epidermis thickly covered with hairs. Crusts are not very suitable for further microscopic examination of the samples and influence unfavourably the examination of the culture. Therefore, crusty foci should, at least, be partly cleared of crusts. Then, parts of the epidermis can be collected from the edge of the affected focus, trying to avoid the bleeding bottom of the crusts.

Material should be collected only from fresh and untreated foci. When samples are available only from lesions treated locally with antimycotics, these places should be cleansed with soap and water or alcohol-ether and the collection of samples should follow — whenever possible — within 2 days.

Areas, where the fungus has penetrated the healthy skin and has started to multiply in it intensively (at the margins of the area), have been found most suitable for demonstrating the presence of the dermatophyte by microscopic examination and cultivation. Usually, less fungal elements are found in the centre of the lesion; their appearance is often changed by various factors (degeneration, disintegration, the influence of defense mechanisms of the attacked organism). Hairs should be removed with the follicles because of the heavy concentration of parasitic elements in these parts. In some cases, Wood's lamp can be useful for selecting hairs suitable for examination. This lamp is the source of ultraviolet light of about 3,650 Å, filtered through the so-called Wood filter, containing nickel oxide. Hairs attacked by some fungi and viewed under the rays of this lamp in a dark room fluoresce in yellow-green or green-blue colours. This fluorescence is particularly valuable for the detection of microspora and, therefore, suitable for collecting hairs from small animals. However, the absence of fluorescence never excludes the possibility of dermatophytic infection and this method should be considered only as auxiliary.

Exudate and pus can be transferred from vesicular or pustular efflorescences with bacteriological needles directly into the media. Hair and scale samples can be cultivated successfully for several weeks or even months after collection and used for repeated and longlasting microscopical examination. Cotton-wool tampons are not suitable because the fungal elements, adhering to them, cannot be kept for any length of time. In addition, moist tampons render a perfect breeding ground for contaminating moulds and bacteria.

When collecting materials from suspected dermal lesions of animals and storing them in glass containers, these should be kept absolutely dry. Increased humidity supports germination of saprophytic spores and hampers further examination of the samples. For the same reason the use of rubber stoppered glass tubes cannot be recommended. Each sample tube should be labelled as mentioned in the foregoing text and accompanied by a request form for the examining laboratory including data on the animal species, the name of the locality, the name of the owner, the attending veterinarian, the course of infection and other data of importance (e.g. medical treatment, epizootological data etc.). There should be sufficient samples available for repeated examination.

For collecting samples of hairs and epidermal scales from animals with no gross clinical symptoms (latent dermatophytosis) Mackenzie's hair-brush technique (MACKENZIE 1963) may be used. In this case, the fur of the animals is combed with sterile brushes or metal combs. The combed out hairs fall either directly into the dish with the cultivation medium or are collected and placed into sterile petri dishes. Microscopical examination and cultivation follows later. After using either comb or brush, the media can be inoculated by pressing the teeth of the comb or the bristles of the brush into the dish with the medium. Used brushes can be placed separately into sterile paper bags and taken to a more distant laboratory for further examination. The material obtained (hairs on the brushes etc.) can also be studied under filtered ultra-violet radiation (Wood's light) and only fluorescing hairs selected for further examination.

Collection of keratinous material from claws and hoofs will not be described in detail. Dermatophytic infections of these appendages are not very frequent in animals (dogs, cats). For microscopical and cultivation demonstration of the causative agent of onychomycosis, minute parts of a pathologically affected nail are needed; these can be scraped off with a sharp glass slide, an old scalpel or a dental drill.

When collecting specimens, all necessary precautions should be observed (gloves, overalls, rubber aprons, thorough disinfection of hands after work). Also all instruments used should be thoroughly disinfected.

III. MICROSCOPICAL EXAMINATION OF SPECIMENS

A prerequisite of the microscopical finding of parasitic fungi in skin scales, hairs etc. is the clearing of the keratinous structures of these materials (hydrolysis of keratinous substances contained in the dermis and its appendages). The following clearing solutions may be used:

20% KOH

For microscopical examination of epidermal scales, crusts, hyperkeratotic masses, keratinous substances from claws and hoofs a. o. This solution is not suitable for clearing hairs, because its softening and decomposing effect causes dispersion of the dermatophytic elements. It should not be used for the diagnosis of nondermatophytic agents in superficial mycoses, e.g. *Candida* species (formation of false, artificial spherical structures, which may be mistaken for yeast-like cells). In this concentration, 20% KOH clears the material after $1/_2$—1 hr. Only fresh solution should be applied.

5% KOH

For microscopical examination of the same material, but the specimens take longer to clear (15—20 hrs). It is of advantage in mass examination, when the preparations can be made on the one day and read on the other.

A better representation of the dermatophytic elements in the specimens can be achieved by adding 10% Parker's blue to potassium hydroxyde solu-

tions (Parker's super chrome blue-black ink from The Parker Pen Co., Janes-
ville, Wisconsin, U.S.A.). The reagent can be kept for about one month.

Potassium hydroxyde with glycerine

Potassium hydroxyde	5·0 g
Glycerine	25·0 g
Distilled water	100·0 ml

The mounting fluid is suitable for clearing epidermal scales and crusts, but
it takes a few hours before the material becomes ready for microscopical
examination.

Aman's lactophenol with cotton blue

Phenol crystals	20·0 g
Lactic acid	20·0 g
Glycerine	40'0 g
Cotton blue	0·05 g
Distilled water	20·0 ml

Aman's chloral lactophenol

Chloral hydrate	2·0 g
Phenol crystals	1·0 g
Lactic acid	1·0 g

Specimens treated with these solutions are ready for examination after a few
minutes. Especially suitable for microscopical examination of hairs. The
preparations can be stored for a considerable length of time.

A mixture containing polyvinylalcohol (KOCH 1963) may be used as
mounting fluid for permanent preparations.

Polyvinylalcohol (of medium viscosity)	10·0 g
Chloral hydrate	20·0 g
Lactic acid	35·0 ml
15% carbolic acid	25.0 ml
Glycerine	10·0 ml
Distilled water	50·0 ml

Specimens treated in potassium hydroxyde or cleared with lactophenol can be
directly transferred into this medium, which dries up very little. Drying up
can be prevented by framing the edges of the cover slip with e.g. Caedax.

For microscopical examination, a drop of any of these fluids is placed
on part of the specimen on a clean slide (a few epidermal scales, hairs) and
a cover slip is added. Large scales or keratinous masses should be grained.
When making preparations from hairs, it is also necessary to view their
follicular part because of the descending tendency of dermatophytic infection
(most elements are found in these parts of the hair).

Although the warming of a preparation over a Bunsen flame has been
recommended by some authors, because it may accelerate the hydrolysis

of keratinous substances, we have found this procedure not too suitable (formation of crystals intervening with the microscopical examination and destruction of cellular elements). The time to elapse between preparation and examination depends largely on the mounting fluid used (see above).

Cleared specimens are viewed under low power objectives ($\times$ 100) for a general orientation. High power objectives ($\times$ 450) are used, when a suitable site has been selected. Only dry magnification is employed and the greatest possible contrast is aimed at.

IV. CULTIVATION

1. General instructions

In the laboratory, the material obtained in accord with the principles for collecting specimens is divided into three parts: one for microscopical examination, one for cultivation, one for possible re-examination, the latter being kept in a container and placed in a refrigerator to be used for re-examination, if required.

The material for culture is inoculated into inoculation media with heat-sterilized and cooled wire loops or needles. Only small particles of the material (single hairs, epidermal scales) should be transferred into the media, the larger ones should be grained before inoculation. The individual inoculates are separately placed into some sites of the agar, either directly on the surface or slightly submerged. A petri dish is more suitable for observing the inoculated area than slants and therefore recommended for veterinary cultivation. On a larger area of culture medium, where the individual colonies are more widely dispersed, there is less danger for the dermatophytic colonies to become rapidly overgrown by contaminants. Secondary contamination and desiccation of the inoculated media may be prevented by covering the dishes with cellophane.

Serous fluid from vesicles or pus from pustules are inoculated into the agar surface by moving the inoculation needle through the agar surface in wavy movements. Before inoculation, the agar plates should be dried in the incubator at 37°C for 15 min to dispose of condensation water, which makes cultivation of separate colonies impossible. Before incubation, the inoculated agar plates should be labelled with the same examination number, under which the examination has been entered into the request form and the log book; the date of inoculation must be added.

It is necessary to inoculate at least two agar plates with a sample of each material. The probability of isolating the dermatophytic agent is increasing with the number of cultivations performed (series examination).

At the present, a number of basic and identifying media are used in myco-logical cultivation techniques. Their choice depends on the experiences ob-tained in the various laboratories. As for ourselves, we shall discuss only such cul-ture media, which have been repeatedly verified in our laboratory and are there in standard use.

2. Media for primary isolation

The medium with an antibacterial and selectively antifungal antibiotic should be employed for isolating the agent of an animal dermatophytosis in primary culture. Even after removing parts of the bacterial and fungal contaminants during primary decontamination of the material, there is still such abundance of undesirable flora on a veterinary sample, inoculated on media without the addition of antibiotics, that an early isolation of suspect colonies of a derma-tophyte is almost impossible. In addition to bacteria and saprophytic mould-like fungi, a number of yeast-like fungi, nocardiae and streptomycetes are also present in such media. Although the most frequent contaminants are known to be some rapidly growing species of fungi — predominantly *Phycomycetes* — the presence of even a single bacterial contaminant makes germination and further growth of the dermatophyte, which is often very slow in its develop-ment, almost impossible. There is one more risk with saprophytic fungi: a less experienced diagnostician may regard them to be dermatophytes (particularly in the earlier stages of growth), thus obtaining false positive results of cultiva-tion in the final evaluation.

The basic medium used for primary cultures is Sabouraud's dextrose agar with cycloheximide (= Actidion, an antibiotic isolated from *Streptomyces griseus* — The Upjohn Company, Kalamazoo, Michigan, U.S.A.) and chlor-amphenicol prepared according to the following formula:*

Bacto-tryptose	10·0 g
Bacto-beef extract	3·0 g
NaCl	5·0 g
Agar	17·0 g
Distilled water ad	1,000·0 ml

Dissolve slowly by heating to boiling point and add:

Dextrose	20·0 g
Yeast extract	3·0 g
Thiamine	0·05 g
Chloramphenicol	0·05 g
Actidione	0·5 g

---

*   Sabouraud's cycloheximide-chloramphenicol medium is commercially produced under the name of Mycosel Agar by Baltimore Biological Co. or Mycobiotic Agar by Difco Co.

Chloramphenicol is dissolved in 10 ml of 70% alcohol and added to the boiling medium, which has to be cooled immediately. Actidione solution (in 10 ml acetone) is added after mixing the medium. After a thorough stirring the medium is distributed into petri dishes.

The amount of cycloheximide given in the directives equals the dose which does not inhibit growth of any of the dermatophytes cultured. In this case, the medium cannot be used for isolation of nondermatophytic agents of superficial animal mycoses (e.g. *Cryptococcus* and *Candida* species); their growth becomes clearly inhibited by this antibiotic. When the causative role of these agents is suspected, other cultures should be made on Sabouraud's dextrose agar without cycloheximide. Neither macro- nor micromorphological characters of the culture are changed by the cycloheximide medium (AJELLO et al. 1963).

Bacterial flora may also be suppressed by adding penicillin (20 units/ml) and streptomycin (40 μg/ml) using these instead of chloramphenicol.

Sabouraud's dextrose agar with desertomycin (a Hungarian antibiotic obtained from *Streptomyces flavofungini*) may also be employed when culturing agents of veterinary dermatophytoses. Before adding it to the medium, desertomycin (50 μg/ml medium) must be dissolved in a small amount of warm distilled water. Although this antibiotic with its marked selective, antifungal properties inhibits also the growth of some microbes (principally cocci) chloramphenicol should be added to the medium in the prescribed amount. Sabouraud's dextrose agar modified with desertomycin proves particularly useful in primary isolation of *Trichophyton verrucosum*. Contrary to cycloheximide it does not inhibit the growth of yeast-like microorganisms of the genus *Candida*.

Some authors (e.g. KIELSTEIN 1963) recommend fungicidin as a selective antifungal antibiotic for primary isolation of dermatophytes. This antibiotic is added to Sabouraud's dextrose agar in an amount of 100—200 μg/l ml. Dimethylformamide in an amount not exceeding 1% of total volume of the medium is employed as a solvent of fungicidin.

Before placing the inoculated and labelled plates in the thermostat, all are wrapped in cellophane, which has been soaked in a weak solution of disinfectant. This precaution is taken against rapid desiccation and secondary air contamination. The petri dishes are also wrapped in cellophane (cut in squares to the size of the dishes — for a 10 cm dia dish a cellophane square of 14 × 14 cm). The cellophane squares are soaked in a 0·5% Ajatin Spofa solution* (solutio aquosa dimethyllaurylbenzylammonii bromati). Then the dishes are tightly covered with lids and incubated either in the incubator at

---

*   Ajatin-Spofa is a Czechoslovak product, but any other similar disinfectant may be used.

27 °C or in the room at room temperature. In the latter case, they must be shaded against direct sunrays. However, an incubator should be used whenever available, because the optimal temperatures for growth of most agents of veterinary dermatophytoses are ranging from 25—30 °C.

3. Isolation

In primary culture, the first signs of growth of the dermatophytes occur mostly between the 4th and 12th day of incubation. From the 4th day onwards, the plates with the inoculated material should be examined regularly every day. Should suspect colonies of a dermatophytic character start to grow from the inoculated parts of the material and no colonies of contaminants found to be present (these may often be recognized by their distinct yellow, green or gray pigmentation) there is no need to isolate the suspect colonies from the plates. Primary cultures of most dermatophytes display such characteristic features that, in most instances, the species can be identified by micromorphological examination.

If contaminants are present in the culture medium, the suspect colonies must be isolated as soon as possible (subcultivation).

Isolation is necessary when the isolate cannot be identified from the primary culture or when the isolated strain has to be preserved (collection of cultures).

Petri dishes with growing cultures have to be handled with great care: vehement movements, causing the spores to spread over the medium, must be avoided to forego an undesirable dispersion of contaminants or spores of the causative agent and the development of atypical colonies.

For identification of the isolate in subcultures, further diagnostic procedures have to be performed. The first requirement is work with a pure culture. To prevent further contamination of the subculture, strictly aseptic conditions have to be observed in isolation and all other manipulation with the culture media. Therefore, subcultures are made on slants in a room sterilized by an UV emitter, on disinfected tables with all windows and ventilations closed.

4. Media for subcultures

Subcultures can be made on Sabouraud's dextrose agar without antibiotics:

Dextrose	30·0 g
Pepton	10·0 g
NaCl	5·0 g
Agar	30·0 g
Distilled water ad	1,000·0 ml

The medium is distributed into tubes, twice sterilized in the Arnold sterilizer and allowed to solidify in slanting position.

Subcultures can also be made on cycloheximide medium.

When transferring isolates, a small portion is removed from the edge of a primary isolated colony with a flame-sterilized and cooled inoculating needle and placed on the surface of a culture medium in a test tube. It should be avoided to inoculate the thinnest agar layer (danger of early desiccation) and care should be taken to keep the test tubes completely free of condensation water, which may cause the spores to spread over the whole agar surface and prevent the isolative manner of inoculation. After opening the test tube and performing the proper inoculation, the margin of the test tube and the stopper are singed with the flame of a Bunsen burner.

Should no suspect colonies be found in primary isolation after three weeks following the inoculation of the material, the culture is considered to be negative. In routine diagnostics, the final evaluation of a positive culture is possible even after this period especially when identification is made from a primary culture. For slowly growing cultures or those which require further diagnostic procedures for identification, the final evaluation should be made after an accordingly prolonged period.

5. Special media

For a reliable identification of a strain grown in primary culture it is necessary to overcome several obstacles. The most frequent is the atypical macromorphological appearance of the isolate or lack of micromorphologically differentiated features in the culture. In both cases, the strain should be subcultured on special media to obtain a more typical manifestation of macromorphological features (character of colony growth, pigmentation etc.) or to stimulate the formation of diagnostically important fructifications.

Media selectively stimulating the formation of some pigments are, e.g. cornmeal agar and potato-dextrose agar, used for differentiating *Trichophyton mentagrophytes* from *T. rubrum*.

Cornmeal agar

Cornmeal	40·0 g
Agar	15·0 g
Distilled water ad	1,000·0 ml

Boil cornmeal lightly in 500 ml water for 1 hr and than filter through gauze. Dissolve agar in 500 ml water and mix with cornmeal. Dispense medium into test tubes, autoclave and allow to solidify in slanting position.

Potato-dextrose agar

Potatoes, infusion from	200·0 g
Dextrose	20·0 g
Agar	15·0 g
Distilled water ad	1,000·0 ml

The medium is placed in test tubes, autoclaved for 10 min at 120 °C and allowed to solidify in slanting position.

Spore production of isolates poorly sporulating on basic media can be stimulated by the use of the so-called natural media, e.g. agar with groats, agar with corn flakes or rice grain medium.

Agar with groats

Groats (wheat, barley)	150·0 g
Agar	15·0 g
Distilled water ad	1,000·0 ml

Heat groats slowly in 500 ml water for 30 min, add agar and the remaining water. When dissolved, place medium in test tubes and sterilize twice for 30 min in the Arnold's sterilizer. Allow medium to solidify in slanting position.

Agar with corn flakes

Corn flakes	30·0 g
Agar	20·0 g
Distilled water	1,000·0 ml

Macerate corn flakes in water for 24 hrs. Add agar and heat to 115 °C in the autoclave. Leave to cool; then place medium in test tubes, sterilize for 20 min in the autoclave and allow to solidify in the test tubes in slanting position.

Rice grain medium

Rice grains	10·0 g
Distilled water	50·0 ml

Boil rice in Erlenmeyer flasks in Arnold's sterilizer and distribute into test tubes, sterilized in Arnold's sterilizer. Allow medium to solidify in slanting position.

6. Cultivation in increased CO_2 tension

Another way of stimulating sporulation of dermatophytes is their cultivation in increased CO_2 tension. Cultures on petri dishes are placed in an aerostat.

About 15% of air is pumped out by a vacuum pump and replaced by the corresponding amount of CO_2. The cultures are incubated for 2 weeks at 28 °C, refilling carbon dioxide every 4 and 8 days (BALABANOFF and KASAROV 1963). CO_2 accelerates the growth of the culture and intensifies pigment production.

7. Isolation of colonies

When no isolated colonies can be obtained in primary isolation, the inoculum from the typical zone of growth should be suspended in sterile physiological saline, thoroughly emulsified and then streaked with wire loops into the isolation media on plates (streak method). Another method for obtaining isolated colonies is the dilution method: a suspension acquired as described in the foregoing method is diluted by degrees with physiological saline and the different dilutions are poured over the agar surface on the plates. Both methods are suitable for obtaining pure stock cultures.

Single-spore cultures are used in genetical, physiological and biometrical studies. A single-spore isolation can be obtained as follows:

a) with the aid of a single-spore isolator: the isolation can be controlled microscopically by fitting a sterile tube to the low power objective of the microscope ($\times$ 10) and lowering it into the agar to cut out a cylindrical piece of agar containing a single, beforehand chosen spore. After lifting the tube, the agar with the spore is blown out by air pressure (using a small ballon) into the new culture medium;

b) with the aid of a micromanipulator.

V. MACROSCOPIC EXAMINATION OF CULTURES

After a certain incubation period depending on the dermatophytic species, cultures can be examined macroscopically. This examination is based on the study of a number of features (for details see chapter A XII and Tables 8—12).

To ensure an exact macroscopic development of the colonies, the culture medium should not be allowed to desiccate (cellophane covers) and should be incubated continuously at a constant temperature. Most suitable for macroscopic examination are the so-called giant colonies on petri dishes. These are obtained by inoculating a small amount of the inoculum into a single point at the centre of the dish.

The number of macroscopic features of a culture depends on the medium used, on the mode of incubation and on the age of the culture; pigmentation, e.g. may be influenced by the presence of traces in the medium, by illumination during cultivation, by the age of the colony a.o. Therefore, standard procedures should be observed in cultivation and, when comparing the individual isolates, only colonies of the same age should be described, photographed etc.

The determination of the colour of the surface of a colony and its reverse is most subjective and it is useful to compare them with standard colour charts. In this book we used Paclt's colour standards (PACLT 1958).

VI. MICROSCOPIC EXAMINATION OF CULTURES

Microscopic examination of a culture is indispensible in identification techniques. The macromorphological properties of some species of dermatophytes are very similar and it seems almost impossible to identify a species on the grounds of a single analysis of its macroscopic characters.

When studying the micromorphology of a culture, characteristic formations of diagnostic importance can be found, e.g. fructifications (macroconidia, microconidia, asci with ascospores), different types of hyphae (racquets, spirals a. o.). (For details see A XI b.)

1. Preparations in mounting fluids

For microscopic examination, part of the culture is removed with a flame-sterilized inoculation needle from the agar medium, placed on a slide, torn apart with two sterile needles in a drop of Lugol's solution or lactophenol and covered with a cover slip. Most important is the choice of a suitable site: in older cultures, the particle should be taken from the edge of the colony, in young cultures preferably from the centre; sometimes it is advisable to remove the entire circumference of the colony. When failing to find the desired formations in the first preparation, another one should be made from a different part of the colony. Slides and cover slips used for microscopic examination should be clean and clear of all grease. Lugol's solution and lactophenol are used in the first identification of micromorphological properties and in more detailed studies in connection with the size of the elements. If the torn up portion of culture soaks badly in Lugol's solution, it should be dipped in 70% alcohol and then in Lugol's solution.

Instead of Lugol's solution or lactophenol a mixture of glycerol and alcohol can be used for making a microscopic preparation from a culture:

Glycerol	4 parts
Alcohol 96%	2 parts
Distilled water	4 parts

First, the preparation is viewed under a low power microscope and after finding the desired formations, a magnification of × 450 is employed. When viewing more detailed structures (the character of the cell membrane of spores etc.), an oil immersion lense is applied.

2. Slide cultures

When studying slide cultures, the micromorphology of a culture (various modes of the development of the reproductive organs a. o.) can be traced during the different periods of the colony's growth. Some methods for the preparation of slide cultures are given in the following text:

a) Unstained slide cultures

Test tubes with melted Sabouraud's agar (temperatures not exceeding 45—50°C) are massively inoculated with pure culture and well stirred with a sterile glass rod. A drop of inoculated agar is transferred to a slide lying on a U-shaped glass rod at the bottom of a petri dish. The drop of still liquid agar is covered with a slip the opposite edges of which are resting on cover slips. Then about 5 ml distilled water is added to the dish to prevent desiccation of the culture. The dishes are covered with lids and incubated at 27°C. Slides, cover slips, U-shaped glass rods,. petri dishes and distilled water are sterilized before use. After 3—5 days of incubation, the slides with the growing cultures are removed from the dishes and the cultures are viewed under the microscope. Microscopic examination is continued for the duration of culture growth.

b) Slide cultures stained with cotton blue (AJELLO et al. 1963).

Agar blocks 10 × 10 mm from plates of Sabouraud's dextrose agar are placed under sterile condition at a height of 2—3 mm on slides lying on U-shaped glass rods at the bottom of the petri dishes. Only sterile glass ware should be used. The culture is inoculated into the centre of each of the four sides of the agar block square and covered with a coverslip. After moistening the bottom of the petri dishes with 8 ml of sterile water, the dishes are incubated at 25°C. When sporulation appears, the coverslip is removed from the block and placed, face downwards, into a drop of lactophenol cotton blue on a new slide, whereby care should be taken to keep the growing culture on the slide, when removing the agar block from the original slide. Then, another drop of lactophenol cotton blue and a new coverslip is placed on the culture; excessive liquid has to be swapped off from the preparations before framing them with asphalt tar varnish. Such preparations can be used as permanent mounts.

VII. OTHER DIAGNOSTIC METHODS

Sometimes it is impossible to identify reliably the dermatophyte species only by its morphological characters. Therefore, additional diagnostic tests should be performed should there be any doubt about the identity of the species (atypical strains; strains, similar in their characteristic signs to those found in a number of other dermatophytes). In view of the specific physiological properties of dermatophytes it is possible to use, for instance, methods investigating metabolic activites of some species. Nutritional tests and the tests of keratinolytic activity in vitro are important in the diagnostic practice. Both methods are employed mainly for identifying species of the genus *Trichophyton*.

1. Nutritional tests

are based on the fact that some species of dermatophytes exhibit specific metabolic requirements for some vitamins or amino-acids which they cannot synthetize. Therefore, they fail to grow on media containing casein or ammonium nitrate only. E. g. *Trichophyton equinum* strictly requires nicotinic acid, *T. megninii* l-histidine. In this they differ from all other dermatophytes. Growth of *T. tonsurans* is stimulated by adding thiamine, thus distinguishing it from *T. mentagrophytes*, *T. rubrum* etc.

Casein agar and ammonium nitrate agar are employed for stock media in the above tests.

Casein agar

Casein, 10% acid hydrolyzed, vitamin-free	25·0 ml
Glucose	40·0 g
$MgSO_4$	0·1 g
KH_2PO_4	1·8 g
Agar	20·0 g
Dist. water q. s.	1,000·0 ml

After dissolving the medium by heating, it is distributed into Erlenmeyer flasks (100 ml per flask) and autoclaved for 15 min at 120 °C. Part of the medium is dispensed into test tubes to be used in vitamin-free control, the rest of the medium is used as a basis for further media.

Ammonium nitrate agar

1·5 g NH_4NO_3 substitutes the casein, the rest of the formula remains unchanged (see casein agar).

Stock vitamin solution

Thiamine solution

Thiamine hydrochloride	1·0 mg
Dist. water	100·0 ml

Inositol solution

i-inositol	250·0 mg
Dist. water	100·0 ml

Histidine solution

l-histidine	150·0 mg
Dist. water	100·0 ml

Nicotinic acid solution

Nicotinic acid	10·0 mg
Dist. water	100·0 ml

All these vitamin solutions are autoclaved at 120°C/10 min and stored in the refrigerator.

Test media

Thiamine-casein agar, inositol-casein and nicotinic acid-casein agar are prepared by adding 2 ml stock vitamin solution to 100 ml melted casein agar. The medium is distributed into test tubes, sterilized and slanted.

In the preparation thiamine-inositol-casein agar solutions of both vitamins (2 ml each) are added to 100 ml melted casein agar.

When preparing histidine-ammonium nitrate agar, 2 ml stock solution of histidine are added to 100 ml melted ammonium nitrate agar. The medium is distributed into test tubes, sterilized and slanted.

Test tubes with nutrition media should be inoculated with only one small particle of the investigated culture (the size of a pin head) to avoid transferring the not vitamin-free medium on which the strain was cultured. The results of these tests are shown on Table 19. In each group we have listed such pairs and triads of species, which are morphologically similar and may be mistaken for another species.

The capability of growth in *T. concentricum*, *T. schoenleinii* and *T. verrucosum* has been estimated after an incubation of the strains lasting 7—14 days at 37°C, for the other species after 7—10 days of incubation at room temperature.

2. Study of the manner of growth in liquid media

Liquid media may also be used for identifying some dermatophytes. To differentiate *T. mentagrophytes* from *T. rubrum*, the growth properties may be tested in a 10% peptone solution (REFAI, RIETH and ITO 1964).

Peptone	10·0 g
Dist. water	100·0 ml

The pH is adjusted to 6·4, bromthymol blue is used as indicator. The solution is distributed into test tubes and repeatedly treated in Arnold's sterilizer. The tubes are inoculated with a small portion of the investigated culture and incubated at room temperature.

T. mentagrophytes always grows on the surface of the solution in light brown colonies with depressions and craters.

T. rubrum grows either on the surface of the solution in snow-white, cottony, hemispherical colonies or submerged into the solution.

3. Hair perforation test

Keratinolytic activity of the individual dermatophyte species can be studied on hair culture in vitro.

Hairs of man and of various mammals (e. g. mouse, guinea-pig, dog, sheep, horse) are used in this test. The cut hairs are thoroughly washed and rinsed in distilled water. After drying at room temperature they are sterilized in petri dishes in an autoclave (1·2 atm. 20 min). Hairs of short-haired animals are used directly, hairs of man and sheep are cut into pieces 1·5 to 2 cm in length. Then they are spread over a petri dish in 10 ml sterile distilled water with 2 drops of sterile 10% yeast extract and inoculated with the investigated culture. At the end of a fortnight's incubation at 27 °C, single hairs or their segments are removed from the dish, placed on a slide and cleared in a drop of lactophenol before being examined under the microscope to estimate the mode of perforation or destruction of the hair (Table 18). Microscopic examination of the hair culture is repeated after a fortnight.

VIII. EXPERIMENTAL INOCULATION OF ANIMALS

Laboratory animals may be experimentally inoculated with both dermatophytic cultures and with material taken from the examined lesions (hairs, epidermal scales). This experimental inoculation of a culture is used for additional diagnostic methods: the capability of producing dermatophytosis, the character of the provoked lesion and especially the type of parasitism of the hairs in vivo helps in reliable identification of the isolated strain. Also vital passages may be used for "reviving" a strain kept for too long on artificial media. Inoculation of material from examined specimens is exceptional and performed only when a highly contaminated sample makes it impossible to reveal the causative agent by cultivation.

Generally guinea-pigs are used for experimental infection, but also laboratory mice, rats, rabbits, cats and large domestic animals (e.g. horses). Susceptibility in animals of the same species has been found to vary and therefore, 2—3 animals must be infected with the same strain. Although a dependence of the course of experimental infection on the pigmentation of the hairs has not been proved, pathological changes can be better evaluated on albinos.

1. Inoculation of culture

Hairs are carefully cut off from the abdominal region or the flanks (an area of about 5 × 5 cm) of the experimental animal; if the animal is bigger, also from other sites. Hairs can also be removed by shaving, depilation etc., whereby the epidermis should never be damaged. The site of inoculation is washed with warm water and left to dry. The inoculate of a culture is swabbed onto the skin slightly scarified with emery paper (bleeding must be avoided). For the inoculation proper either a thick suspension of the culture in physiological saline or some part of the culture mixed with a few drops of honey is used. The inoculate is swabbed on a sterile glass rod, wire loop etc.

Two to three days after inoculation, a light traumatic reaction, redness at the site of inoculation can be observed in most of the animals. A week later, the site is usually edematous and exudate starts to ooze through the skin, which is then changing into whitish or yellowish crusts. Sometimes the process is of an infiltrating nature causing deep necroses and affections which heal into scars. Hairs, as a rule, are afflicted at a later stage. Slightly pathogenic strains cause the occurrence of erythematosquamous patches, healing spontaneously soon after. Some dermatophytes may even produce scutula.

Material for microscopical examination and cultivation may be obtained from well developed lesions. Sometimes, the inoculated dermatophyte can be recultivated from the site of inoculation even if lesions fail to develop.

The result of the test may be affected by the age of the culture used. Therefore, younger, 3—4 week-old cultures are preferred in experimental infection. "Florentiform" strains with numerous aerial spores usually exhibit a marked pathogenicity. Inoculation of strains growing in "glabrous" colonies is generally not very successful.

2. Inoculation of a sample of clinical material

is similar to the foregoing procedure. The inoculum is prepared by mixing hairs, epidermal scales etc. with a small amount of Sabouraud's dextrose agar and rubbing it into the scarified skin.

IX. INDUCTION OF PERFECT STATES

Longlasting cultivation on a mixture of surface soil and hairs is used for inducing perfect states of dermatophytes. Agar media (agar with an admixture of keratin, corn meal agar with dextrose a. o.) are used only for detailed genetic studies. Usually the method of ,,keratinous bait on soil" ("hair-on-soil culture") can be used in the diagnosis of most cases.

Preparation of "hair-on-soil cultures":

Sterile hairs or their segments are mixed on petri dishes with nonsterile soil, free of keratinophilic fungi. The inoculum obtained by scraping the culture is added, or the dishes are inoculated by pipetting a spore-mycelial suspension to the hairs. Another way is the use of squares of agar medium (3—5 mm) with a grown culture, placed on a layer of soil in a petri dish (growth facing upwards) and covered with hairs (BENEDEK 1964), keeping the soil sufficiently moist. The dishes are incubated at 24 °C or even less (e.g. *T. terrestre*). — Fruit bodies develop after 10—30 days.

Fruit body formation is stimulated by the presence of microorganisms contained in the soil and by their metabolites. Keratinaceous substances have no stimulating influence (BENEDEK 1964). The type of soil is of no importance, the pH tolerance ranging from 5—8. The best keratinaceous substances have been found in the hairs of horses and children (DAWSON, GENTLES and BROWN 1964). Microcultivation techniques of fruit body formation has been described by HEJTMÁNKOVÁ-UHROVÁ (1966).

X. RESISTANCE OF DERMATOPHYTES

The results of cultivation depends also on the resistance of the dermatophytes. In clinical material, cultures and in nature their resistance varies greatly according to conditions of the external environment. In the laboratory they remain viable in epidermal scales and hairs for 1—2 years (DVOŘÁK, HUBÁLEK, OTČENÁŠEK 1968). Desiccation and preservation at low temperatures are comparatively well tolerated by dermatophytes and they can stand up better to lower than to higher temperature, most of them dying at 50—58 °C. In soil, however, dermatophytes are far more resistant to the effects of temperature than in the laboratory. Radiation kills them within a very short time (20 min) (KAŠKIN 1962).

In garden soil, dermatophytic spores survive for several years. According to SCHÖNBORN (1966) *T. mentagrophytes* was found to survive for 4 years and 8 months, *T. verrucosum* for 9 months. *M. gypseum* was re-isolated from naturally animated soil after 3 years, *T. mentagrophytes* after one year and 10 months. All of them retained their original morphological properties.

In plant material (hay, straw) dermatophytes can survive but their virulence decreases.

XI. STORAGE OF DERMATOPHYTIC CULTURE IN MYCOLOGICAL COLLECTION

1. Maintenance of viable cultures

Often, a viable collection of dermatophytic culture has to be preserved in the laboratory as type specimens, for comparison with less typical isolates etc. The cultures should retain their original macro- and microscopic character. The following methods, having different requirements as to time, range of application etc. may be used for a longlasting preservation of cultures:

Storage of cultures at room temperature

A simple, but time-consuming method requiring transfer of cultures at intervals of 2—3 months. Subcultures are made in test tubes, transferring a typical portion of the colony. Part of the culture becomes pleomorphic if kept too long in the subculture. Desiccation of the medium can be retarded by covering the cotton stopper with cellophane or by sealing the tube with paraffin.

Storage of cultures in lowered temperature

Culture tubes are kept in the refrigerator or a cool room at a temperature of 5—10°C. Cultures desiccate less and are subcultured at intervals of a few months. However, not all dermatophytes can stand up to prolonged storage in lowered temperature. This method is unsuitable for storing e. g. *E. floccosum*, *M. audouinii*, *T. schoenleinii* and *T. violaceum* (AJELLO et al. 1963).

Storage of cultures in the deep-freeze

This is the best method to be used with dermatophytes. 10—14 day-old culture tubes are placed in the deep-freeze at a temperature of about —20°C.

Storage of dermatophytes in "water culture" (CASTELLANI 1960, 1963, BENEDEK 1962)

Culture particles are placed in test tubes or bottles containing 5—10 ml sterile distilled water or physiological saline, stoppered with cotton or rubber stoppers (bottles with screw-tops sterilized for 20 min before use at 120°C). When transferring a culture, no solid medium should be removed with the culture. The cultures in the vessels can be kept for some months at room temperature or in the refrigerator (+5°). After 6—9 months the viability of the cultures is tested (transfer to solid medium) and new subcultures are prepared. This method is useful for the prevention of pleomorphic changes. The dermatophytes retain their characteristic properties even after a year of uninterrupted storage in this environment.

Storage of cultures under a layer of mineral oil

An actively growing culture in a test tube is embedded in sterile mineral oil (sterilisation in Erlenmeyer flasks in the autoclave for 45 min at 120°C). The oil layer must cover the whole surface of the agar and not only the culture. Cultures can be kept viable at room temperature for even several years (AJELLO et al. 1963). Sometimes continued mycelial growth may be observed under the oil layer.

Lyophilization

This method has not proved successful for dermatophytes.

2. Preservation of dead cultures

For preserving only the original macroscopic appearance of a culture (texture of the colony, pigmentation etc.), the tube with the culture is closed with cotton stopper dipped in 4% formalin. Against desiccation the stopper is sealed with paraffin. The culture is killed with formalin vapours, but its macroscopic appearance is preserved in these closed tubes for several years.

3. Benedek's "mycotheca" in lactophenol

To preserve part of the culture for later microscopic examination, lactophenol can be used (BENEDEK 1962). After a certain time a mycotheca, completing the live culture collection and suitable for comparative studies etc., can thus be obtained.

Culture particles are preserved in 15 ml or 30 ml brown bottles with screw caps, filled with lactophenol to one half or three quarters. By immersing the culture into lactophenol, growth can be arrested at any chosen stage. Cultures preserved in this way may be stored for months or even years and re-examined microscopically whenever needed. This method is particularly suitable for storing dermatophytic stages, which are difficult to obtain otherwise (e.g. cleistocarpous perithecia).

Subject:	Age:
bull no 50	2 years

Address:
State farm, Holice 12

Occupation: /

Establishment: /

Clinical diagnosis:	Duration of disease:
trichophytia	2 weeks

Therapy before specimen collection: ø

Specimen collected: hairs and crusts from the head	Date of specimen collection: 22/2 1965
Sender: District veterinary hosp. Pardubice	

Result of microscopical examination: large spores outside the hair	Date of specimen arrival: 23/2 1965

Result of cultivation: T. verrucosum	Date result dispatched: 12/3 1965

Sample card No 1.

Sample card No 2.

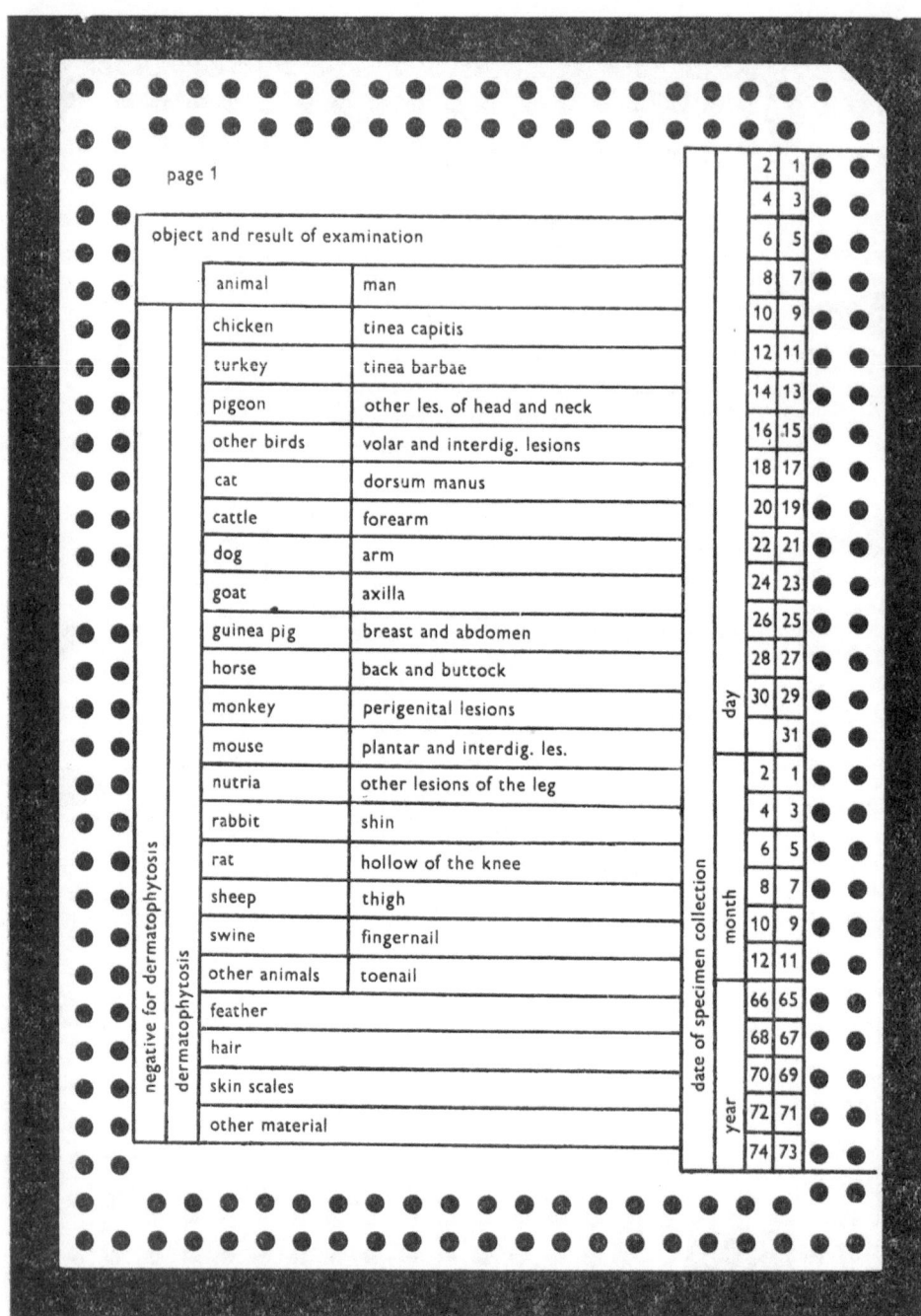

Punching key to card 1.

Punching key to card 2.

XII. INFECTION OF CULTURES BY MITES

Cultures of dermatophytes and of other microscopic fungi can become infected with mites, brought to the laboratory with soil, used for hair baiting, with the air stream etc. Most frequently, these mites belong to the well-known fungus feeding genus *Tarsonemus*. The arthropods can penetrate the cotton stopper of the test tube and destroy the culture completely. A mere transfer of the culture is ineffective because the mites and their eggs are transferred together with the inoculum. Therefore, chemical acaricides must be applied. Most of the drugs recommended in recent years (e.g. para-dichlor-benzene; dichloro-ethane a.o.) are toxic for man and have undesirable fungicidal effects. Therefore, we recommend the following more recent two methods for mite control:

Cultivation on a medium containing lindane (AJELLO et al. 1963)

0·01% lindane powder is added to Sabouraud's dextrose agar or to other standard culture media. After distributing the medium into tubes, it is autoclaved in the usual way. Lindane kills mites in a very short time without affecting the growth of the culture.

Exposure of cultures to thymol fumes (BENEDEK 1963)

The culture is placed on a thin layer of thymol crystals covering the bottom of the tin container or vessel, which are covered. The accumulating thymol fumes kill the adult mites and their eggs. This method is also suitable for removing mites from hair baited soil culture. Thymol fumes are not toxic for man neither by contact nor inhalation.

XIII. RECOMMENDED PROCEDURE FOR THE COLLECTION AND PRESERVATION OF IMPORTANT DATA OBTAINED IN LABORATORY EXAMINATION

In our laboratory we developed and used during the past 15 years a system for the collection and preservation of important data obtained from the results of our examination by entering them on punch cards. In our opinion an analogous system could be used in any laboratory.

For each case examined a card is completed (see sample cards). Only one type of card is used for both animal and human cases. The punching keys are shown on pp. 168 and 169.

In most cases, mycological laboratories are interested in both veterinary and human infection, because animal dermatophytoses are very often transmitted to man and vice versa.

ADDENDUM

Recently, much information has become available which ought to be added to our book. However, for various reasons (lack of space etc.) our choice had to be limited to items which, to some extent, may change our original information. As to taxonomic problems we recommend to replace the term *Microsporon* by *Microsporum,* as suggested by AJELLO (Sabouraudia 6,147—159, 1968). Because his paper contains also various information on new species and proves the validity of older species, we are adding the complete list of AJELLO's classification of imperfect species.

Epidermophyton Sabouraud, 1910
   E. floccosum (Harz, 1870) Langeron et Milochevitch, 1930
Microsporum Gruby 1843
   M. amazonicum Moraes, Borelli et Feo, 1967
   M. audouinii Gruby, 1843
   M. boullardii Dominik et Majchrowicz, 1965
   M. canis Bodin, 1902
   M. cookei Ajello, 1959
   M. distortum Di Menna et Marples, 1954
   M. ferrugineum Ota, 1921
   M. fulvum Uriburu, 1909
   M. gypseum (Bodin, 1907) Guiart et Grigorakis, 1928
   M. nanum Fuentes, 1956
   M. persicolor (Sabouraud, 1910) Guiart et Grigorakis, 1928
   M. praecox Rivalier, 1954
   M. racemosum Borelli, 1965
   M. vanbreuseghemii Georg, Ajello, Friedman et Brinkman, 1962
Trichophyton Malmsten, 1845
   T. ajelloi (Vanbreuseghem, 1952) Ajello, 1968
   T. concentricum Blanchard, 1895
   T. equinum (Matruchot et Dassonville, 1898) Gedoelst, 1902
   T. gallinae (Mégnin, 1881) Silva et Benham, 1952
   T. georgiae Varsavsky et Ajello, 1964

T. gloriae Ajello, 1967

T. gourvilii Catanei, 1933

T. longifusus (Florian et Galgóczy, 1964) Ajello, 1968

T. megninii Blanchard, 1896

T. mentagrophytes (Robin, 1853) Blanchard, 1896

T. phaseoliforme Borelli et Feo, 1966

T. rubrum (Castellani, 1910) Sabouraud, 1911

T. schoenleinii (Lebert, 1845) Langeron et Milochevitch, 1930

T. simii (Pinoy, 1912) Stockdale, Mackenzie et Austwick, 1965

T. soudanense Joyeux, 1912

T. terrestre Durie et Frey, 1957

T. tonsurans Malmsten, 1845

T. vanbreuseghemii Rioux, Jarry et Juminer, 1964

T. verrucosum Bodin, 1902

T. violaceum Bodin, 1902

We are also giving AJELLO's review (1968) of imperfect and corresponding perfect states of species belonging to the imperfect genera *Microsporum* and *Trichophyton* (perfect states: *Nannizzia* and *Arthroderma*):

Perfect state	Imperfect state
Arthroderma	*Trichophyton*
A. benhamiae Ajello et Cheng, 1967	*T. mentagrophytes*
A. ciferrii Varsavsky et Ajello, 1964	*T. georgiae*
A. gertleri Böhme, 1967	*T. vanbreuseghemii*
A. gloriae Ajello, 1967	*T. gloriae*
A. lenticularum Pore, Tsao et Plunkett, 1965	*T. terrestre*
A. quadrifidum Dawson et Gentles, 1961	*T. terrestre*
A. simii Stockdale, Mackenzie et Austwick, 1965	*T. simii*
A. uncinatum Dawson et Gentles, 1961	*T. ajelloi*
Nannizzia	*Microsporum*
N. cajetani Ajello, 1961	*M. cookei*
N. fulva Stockdale, 1963	*M. fulvum*
N. grubyia Georg, Ajello, Friedman et Brinkman, 1962	*M. vanbreuseghemii*
N. gypsea Stockdale, 1963	*M. gypseum*
N. incurvata Stockdale, 1961	*M. gypseum*
N. obtusa Dawson et Gentles, 1961	*M. nanum*
N. persicolor Stockdale, 1967	*M. persicolor*

The list of imperfect species has been completed by two recently described species: *Trichophyton fluviomuniense* (MIGUENS M. P.: Sabouraudia 6, 312—317, 1968) and *T. proliferans* (ENGLISH M. P., STOCKDALE P. M.: Sabouraudia 6, 267—270, 1968).

172

Since we are unable to give a complete list of dermatophytes discovered recently in other countries, we are mentioning only some findings in soil: *Microsporum nanum* — France (COUDERT J., MICHEL-BRUN J., BATTESTI M. R.: Bull. Mens. Soc. Linn., Lyon 36, 187—195, 1967); *M. vanbreuseghemii* — India (AJELLO — personal communication); T. *simii* — India (PADHYE A. A., CARMICHAEL J. W.: Sabouraudia 6, 238—240, 1968).

We should like to add at least some of the recently obtained knowledge on laboratory methods. Also here the choice was extremely difficult.

Lab-lemco media stimulate selectively the formation of dermatophytic pigments and are particularly suitable for differentiating *Trichophyton mentagrophytes* and *T. rubrum* (BAXTER M.: Sabouraudia 3, 72—80, 1963; OTČENÁŠEK M.: Zbl. Bakt. Orig. 206, 550—554, 1968).

Composition of the medium

Lab-lemco beef extract (Oxoid, London)	0·25 %	
Dextrose	0·5 %	
Agar	2·0 %	pH 6·5 — 7·5

After inoculating the medium in the test tubes with the dermatophyte, it is incubated at 27°C. Twelve to 14 days later, pigmentation of the reverse side is evaluated.

T. rubrum: dark rose red

T. mentagrophytes: no colour or dark brown. Biochemical differentiation of *T. mentagrophytes* and *T. rubrum* can be obtained by using the urease test (the splitting of urea) on a modified Christensen's medium (PHILPOT Ch.: Sabouraudia 5, 189—193, 1967; OTČENÁŠEK M.: Zbl. Bakt. Orig. 206, 550—554, 1968).

Composition of the medium

Peptone	1·0 g
NaCl	5·0 g
KH_2PO_4	2·0 g
Dextrose	5·0 g
Agar	20·0 g
Dist. water ad	1,000·0 ml

Dissolve the mixture by heating and add 6 ml of phenol red solution (0.2% in 50% alcohol). Sterilize medium by autoclaving at 115 °C for 15 min, cool to 50 °C and add 100 ml urea (sterile 20% aqueous solution). Dispense medium in test tubes and leave to solidify in slanting position. Inoculate the strain of dermatophyte under investigation onto the surface of the medium, incubate at 27 °C and evaluate results after 8 days. Urease positive strains produce deep red colour throughout the medium (production of an alkaline pH).

T. mentagrophytes: urease present (positive reaction, reddening of the medium), *T. rubrum*: urease absent (negative reaction, colour of medium unchanged).

Table 1
Comparison of three classification systems of dermatophytes

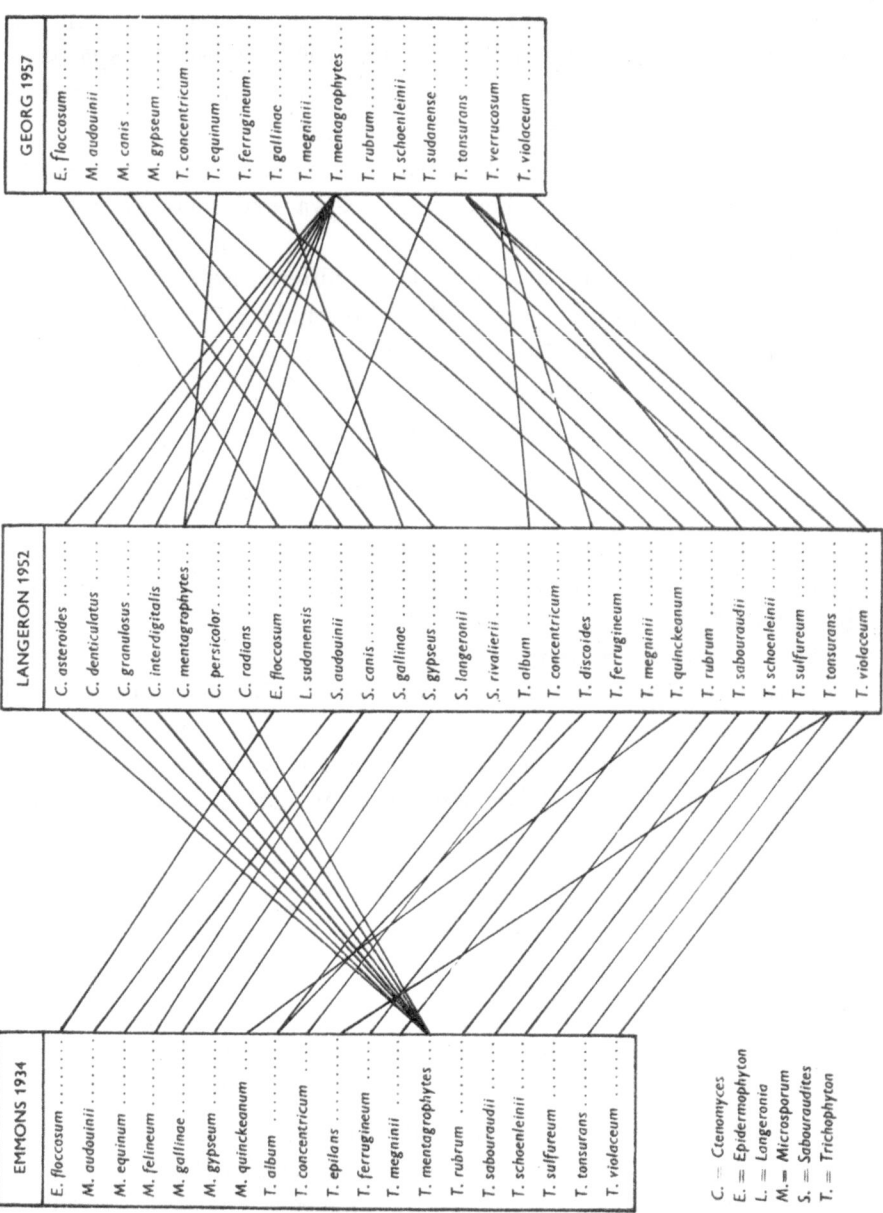

C. = Ctenomyces
E. = Epidermophyton
L. = Langeronia
M. = Microsporum
S. = Sabouraudites
T. = Trichophyton

Table 2

The survey of hosts of dermatophytes

	soil	canary	chicken	turkey	pigeon	sp. unknown	baboon	buffalo	cat	cattle	chinchilla	daman	dog	donkey	dromedary	fox	goat	guinea-pig	hedgehog	horse	kangaroo	lion	monkey	mouse	mule	muskrat	nutria	opossum	polecat	porcupine	rabbit	rat	sheep	squirrel	swine	tapir	tiger	man
E. floccosum										●			●					●		●				●														▲
K. ajelloi	+												▲																									●
K. ajelloi var. *nana*																																						●
M. audouinii																							●●								●							◄
M. canis			●				●		◄	●	●		●	●			●	●		●		●	●								●●		●		●			◄
M. cookei	+																	●													●			●				●
M. distortum																															●							●
M. ferrugineum																																						●
M. fulvum/*M. gypseum*	+									●		●	●					●		●			●	●								●			●◄		●	●	◄
M. nanum	+																																		●			●
M. vanbreuseghemii	+?																																					●
T. concentricum																																						●
T. equinum																				◄																		●
T. gallinae		●	◄	◄	●																																	◄
T. gourvilii			●●																																			●
T. megninii																																						●
T. mentagrophytes	+?		●			●		●	●	●	●		●	●		●	●	●		●	●		●	●	●	●	●	●	●	●	●	●	●	●	●			●
T. mentagrophytes var. *erinacei*	+?																		●◄																			●
T. mentagrophytes var. *interdigitale*	+?																																					▲
T. mentagrophytes var. *quinckeanum*	+?																							◄														▲
T. rubrum													●●																									◄
T. schoenleinii	+?												●											●														◄
T. simii	+?		◄																				◄															◄
T. sudanense	+																																					◄
T. terrestre	+																																					●
T. tonsurans									●				●							●																		●
T. verrucosum		●	●		●			●	●	●●●			●●		●	●	●	●		●●●					●●						●●		●●		●			◄◄
T. violaceum									●	◄			●										●															●●
T. yaoundei																																						◄◄

+ saprophytizes in soil, +? probably saprophytizes in soil, ● host, ▲ important host

175

Table 3

Location of human dermatophytic lesions

	tinea*						
	capitis	barbae	corporis	manus	pedis	cruris	unguium
E. floccosum	(+)	(+)	+	+	++	+++	+
K. ajelloi			+				
K. a. var. *nana*	not reported as the cause of human lesion						
M. audouinii	+++	(+)	+		(+)	(+)	(+)
M. canis	+++	(+)	++		(+)		(+)
M. cookei			+				
M. distortum	+		+				
M. ferrugineum	+++	(+)	+				(+)
*M. fulvum/M. gypseum***	++	+	++		(+)		(+)
M. nanum	+		+				
M. vanbreuseghemii	+						
T. concentricum			+++				(+)
T. equinum	+	+	+				
T. gallinae	+		+			(+)	(+)
T. gourvilii	++		+				
T. megninii	+	+	+				(+)
T. mentagrophytes	+	++	+++	+	+	+	+
T. m. var. *erinacei*			+	+			
T. m. var. *interdigitale*	(+)	(+)	+	+	+++	+	+
T. m. var. *quinckeanum*	+	+	+			(+)	(+)
T. rubrum	(+)	(+)	++	++	+++	++	++
*T. schoenleinii***	++	+	++				+
T. simii				+			
T. sudanense	++		+		(+)		(+)
T. terrestre	not reported as the cause of human lesion						
T. tonsurans	+++	++	++		(+)		(+)
T. verrucosum	+	+	+++		(+)		
*T. violaceum***	+++	(+)	++				(+)
T. yaoundei	++						

* The term "tinea" is the Latin word for worm. It was believed that the round or serpentine-shaped lesions in the skin were caused by worms.

** Sometimes scutula are formed.

Table 4

The distribution of dermatophytes on the Continents

	North America	South America	Africa	Europe	Asia	Australia and/or Oceania
E. floccosum	+	+	+	+	+	+
K. ajelloi	+	+	+	+	+	+
K. a. var. nana				+		
M. audouinii	+	+	+	+	+	+
M. canis	++	+	+	+	+	+
M. cookei	+	+	+	+	+	+
M. distortum	+					+
M. ferrugineum		(+)	+	+	++	
M. fulvum/M. gypseum	+	+	+	+	+	+
M. nanum	+		+			+
M. vanbreuseghemii	+			+		
T. concentricum	+	+			+	++
T. equinum	+	+	?	+	?	+
T. gallinae	+			+		
T. gourvilii			+			
T. megninii			+	+		
T. mentagrophytes	+	+	+	+	+	+
T. m. var. erinacei				+		+
T. m. var. interdigitale	+	+	+	+	+	+
T. m. var. quinckeanum				+		+
T. rubrum	+	+	+	+	+	+
T. schoenleinii	+	+	+	+	+	+
T. simii					+	
T. sudanense	(+)		+	(+)		
T. terrestre	+	+	(+?)	+	+	+
T. tonsurans	+	+	+	(+)	+	+
T. verrucosum	+	+	+	+	+	+
T. violaceum	+	+	+	+	+	+
T. yaoundei			+			

Table 5

Anthropophilic, geophilic and zoophilic dermatophytes and their geographical distribution

Anthropophilic	Geophilic	Zoophilic
exclusively parasitizing man, trichophilic, geographically limited distribution:	exclusively saprophytizing in soil, (probably) world wide distribution:	rarely attacking man, world wide distribution:
M. ferrugineum (Africa, Europe, Asia)	*T. terrestre*	*T. equinum* (horse)
T. gourvilii (Africa)	rarely attacking animals and man, world wide distribution:	*T. gallinae* (birds — hens)
T. sudanense (Africa)	*K. ajelloi*	geographically limited distribution:
T. yaoundei (Africa)	*M. cookei*	*T. simii* (birds?, Asia)
epidermophilic, geographically limited distribution:	geographically limited distribution:	often attacking man, world wide distribution:
T. concentricum (Asia, Oceania, North and South America)	*M. vanbreuseghemii****	*M. canis* (cat, dog)
occasionally attacking animals, trichophilic, world wide distribution:	often attacking animals, rarely man, geographically limited distribution:	*T. mentagrophytes* (rodents?)
M. audouinii	*M. nanum* (pigs, Africa, Australia, North America)	*T. verrucosum* (cattle)
T. schoenleinii	often attacking animals and man, world wide distribution:	geographically limited distribution:
T. tonsurans*	*M. fulvum/gypseum*	*M. distortum***** (cat? Australia, North America)
T. violaceum		
geographically limited distribution:		
T. megninii** (Africa, Europe)		
epidermophilic, pancontinental:		
E. floccosum		
T. rubrum		

* *T. tonsurans* has been reported to cause horse ringworm. However, its similarity to *T. equinum* must be remembered.

** *T. megninii* is by some authors considered to be zoophilic.

*** Till now not isolated from soil, but perfect states known.

**** Anthropophilic?

Table 6

The fluorescence of invaded hairs under the Wood's light

E. floccosum	(does not attack hairs)
K. ajelloi	no fluorescence, only few cases studied
K. a. var. *nana*	(isolated only from soil)
M. audouinii	bright yellow-greenish fluorescence
M. canis	bright yellow-greenish fluorescence
M. cookei	no fluorescence, in rare cases studied
M. distortum	bright yellow greenish fluorescence
M. ferrugineum	bright yellow greenish fluorescence
M. fulvum/M. gypseum	no fluorescence or very poor fluorescence
M. nanum	no fluorescence or very poor fluorescence
M. vanbreuseghemii	no fluorescence or very poor fluorescence
T. concentricum	(does not attack hairs)
T. equinum	no fluorescence
T. gallinae	no fluorescence, only few cases studied
T. gourvilii	no fluorescence
T. megninii	no fluorescence
T. mentagrophytes	no fluorescence
T. m. var. *erinacei*	no fluorescence, only few cases studied
T. m. var. *interdigitale*	(does not attack hairs)
T. m. var. *quinckeanum*	sometimes of greenish fluorescence
T. rubrum	no fluorescence
T. schoenleinii	usually no fluorescence, occasionally gray-whitish or bright yellow-greenish
T. simii	vivid green fluorescence observed several times
T. sudanense	no fluorescence
T. terrestre	does not attack animals or man
T. tonsurans	no fluorescence
T. verrucosum	no fluorescence
T. violaceum	no fluorescence
T. yaoundei	no fluorescence

Table 7

The modes of hair invasion by dermatophytes in vivo

	Main animal host		Man	
	fungus elements			
	inside	outside	inside	outside
	the hair			
E. floccosum	does not attack hair			
K. ajelloi	geophilic, exceptionally attacking animals and man			
K. a. var. nana	isolated only from soil			
M. audouinii	rarely attacks animals*		H	AM 2−3 μm
M. canis	cat, dog*			
M. cookei	geophilic, exceptionally attacking animals and man			
M. distortum	small number of animal infections studied*			AM 2−3 μm
M. ferrugineum	does not attack animals			
M. fulvum/M. gypseum	a wide scale of animals occasionally attacked***		H	ACHI 5−8 μm***
M. nanum	pig	hair invasion not described		ACHI 5−8 μm**
M. vanbreuseghemii	small number of animal infections studied*			ACHI 5−8 μm
T. concentricum	does not attack hair			
T. equinum	horse	H	ACHI large	ACHI
T. gallinae	gallinaceous birds	small number of hairy animal infections studied*	H	A small to large
T. gourvilii	does not attack animals		ACH	ø
T. megninii	rarely attacks animals*			ACHI large
T. mentagrophytes	a wide scale of animals occasionally attacked*		H	ACHI 3−5 μm
T. m. var. erinacei	hedgehog			A small
T. m. var. interdigitale	does not attack hair			
T. m. var. quinckeanum	mouse?	H	S	ACHI small***
T. rubrum	rarely attacks animals		H	ACHI**
T. schoenleinii	a wide scale of animals occasionally attacked			S
T. simii	gallinaceous birds	small number of hairy animal studied	not reported	
T. sudanense	does not attack animals		ACH	ø
T. terrestre	geophilic, not attacking animals and man			
T. tonsurans	rarely attacks animals*		ACH 4 −7.5 μm	ø
T. verrucosum	cattle	H	ACHI 5−10 μm	H · ACHI 5−10 μm
T. violaceum	a wide scale of animals occasionally attacked		ACH 4 −7.5 μm	ø***
T. yaoundei	does not attack animals		ACH 2.7−7.3 μm	ø

   * Animal hair invaded similarly as human.

  ** Sometimes arthrospores inside the hair reported.

*** Sometimes scutula around the hair reported.

A — arthrospores
H — hyphae
M — mosaic-like arrangement of arthrospores forming a sheath
S — scutulum
CH — in chains
I — irregular

Table 8

The ground plan of dermatophyte colonies

	Regular		Irregular		
	circular	asteroid	asteroid	polygonal	lobulate
E. floccosum	+	+			
K. ajelloi	+	+			
K. a. var. *nana*	+				
M. audouinii	+	+			
M. canis	+	+			
M. cookei	+	+			
M. distortum	+	+			
M. ferrugineum	+	+	+	+	+
M. fulvum/M. gypseum	+	+			
M. nanum	+	+	+		
M. vanbreuseghemii	+	+			
T. concentricum	+	+		+	+
T. equinum	+	+			
T. gallinae	+	+		+	
T. gourvilii	+	+	+		
T. megninii	+	+		+	
T. mentagrophytes	+	+			
T. m. var. *erinacei*	+	+			
T. m. var. *interdigitale*	+				
T. quinckeanum	+	+	+	+	
T. rubrum	+				
T. schoenleinii	+	+	+	+	+
T. simii		+			
T. sudanense	+	+	+		+
T. terrestre	+	+			
T. tonsurans	+	+		+	
T. verrucosum	+	+	+	+	+
T. violaceum	+	+		+	+
T. yaoundei	+	+	+	+	+

181

Table 9

The texture of dermatophyte colonies

	Membranous			Filamentous			Granular		Submerged
	glabrous waxy	slightly powdered	filamentous	velvety	fluffy	velvety powdered	finely	coarsely	large submerged mycelium zone on the periphery
E. floccosum						++	+++	+	(+)
K. ajelloi						++		++	
K. a. var nana									
M. audouinii				+	++		+	+	
M. canis					++				(+)
M. cookei			+		+			+	
M. distortum			+	+		+++	++		+
M. ferrugineum	+	+							
M. fulvum/M. gypseum				+		++	+		
M. nanum		+							
M. vanbreuseghemii							+	++	+
T. concentricum			+	++	+	+			
T. equinum									
T. gallinae				+					+
T. gourvilii									
T. megninii							++	++	
T. mentagrophytes	+	+		++	+	++			
T. m. var. erinacei									
T. m. var. interdigitale				+					
T. m. var. quinckeanum							(+)	(+)	
T. rubrum					+	+			
T. schoenleinii			+						
T. simii							++		
T. sudanense		(+)	(+)						
T. terrestre									
T. tonsurans				++			+		
T. verrucosum						++			
T. violaceum	+++	+++	+++						
T. yaoundei									++

182

Table 10

The tendency to form furrows and folds

	Without furrows	Some radial shallow furrows present	Wrinkled or folded
E. floccosum		+	+
K. ajelloi	+	+	
K. a. var. nana	+		
M. audouinii	+	+	
M. canis		+	
M. cookei	+	+	
M. distortum		+	
M. ferrugineum		+	+
M. fulvum/M. gypseum	+	+	
M. nanum		+	
M. vanbreuseghemii	+		
T. concentricum			+
T. equinum	+	+	+
T. gallinae	+	+	+
T. gourvilii			+
T. megninii		+	+
T. mentagrophytes	+	+	
T. m. var. erinacei	+		
T. m. var. interdigitale	+		
T. m. var. quinckeanum		+	+
T. rubrum	+		
T. schoenleinii			+
T. simii	+		
T. sudanense			+
T. terrestre	+		
T. tonsurans			+
T. verrucosum	+		+
T. violaceum			+
T. yaoundei	+		+

Table 11 The surface colour

Colour	E. floccosum	K. ajelloi	K. a. var. nana	M. audouinii	M. canis	M. cookei	M. distortum	M. ferrugineum	M. fulvum/M. gypseum	M. nanum	M. vanbreuseghemii	T. concentricum	T. equinum	T. gallinae	T. gourvilii	T. megninii	T. mentagrophytes	T. m. var. erinacei	T. m. var. interdigitale	T. m. var. quinckeanum	T. rubrum	T. schoenleinii	T. simii	T. sudanense	T. terrestre	T. tonsurans	T. verrucosum	T. violaceum	T. yaoundei
white to grey	●	●	●	●	●	●	●	●	●	●	●	●	●	●		●	●	●	●		●	●	●	●	●	●	●	●	●
pale rosy				●	●	●					●		●					●	●		●	●							
rosy					●	●							●			●			●		●	●							
vinaceous												●										●!							
reddish												●		●															
red												●		●															
blood red												●																	
carmine												●																	
dark blood red																											●		
salmon				●	●	●	●	●	●	●	●		●			●	●				●	●		●	●	●	●	●	●
apricot	●							●	●		●		●					●							●		●		
saffron yellow	●	●											●																
orange	●												●																
terra-cotta								●	●			●																	
rusty								●				●																	
pale lemon yellow		●	●	●	●!	●	●					●!	●			●	●	●	●		●	●	●	●		●	●	●	●
lemon yellow					●!							●														●	●		
yellow							●					●!	●																
egg-yolk-yellow	●!																												
pale yellow greenish	●						●														●		●						
yellow greenish																													
pale violaceous				●																								●	
pale lavender																												●	
lavender																												●	
violaceous																												●	
violet														●														● (brownish)	
lilac				●	●						●		●	●	●				●	●									
pale purplish													●																
mallow purple													●							●									
purplish																				●								●	
purple																												●	
dark purple																												●	
livid purple																												●	
purplish grey																												●	
purplish black																												●	

Additional notations within the table: "white to violet" (T. gallinae / T. gourvilii region), "white to creamy" (T. m. var. erinacei / interdigitale region), "pale buff" (T. schoenleinii region), "brownish" (T. violaceum, violet row).

! pigment diffusing into the medium

184

Table 12

The reverse colour

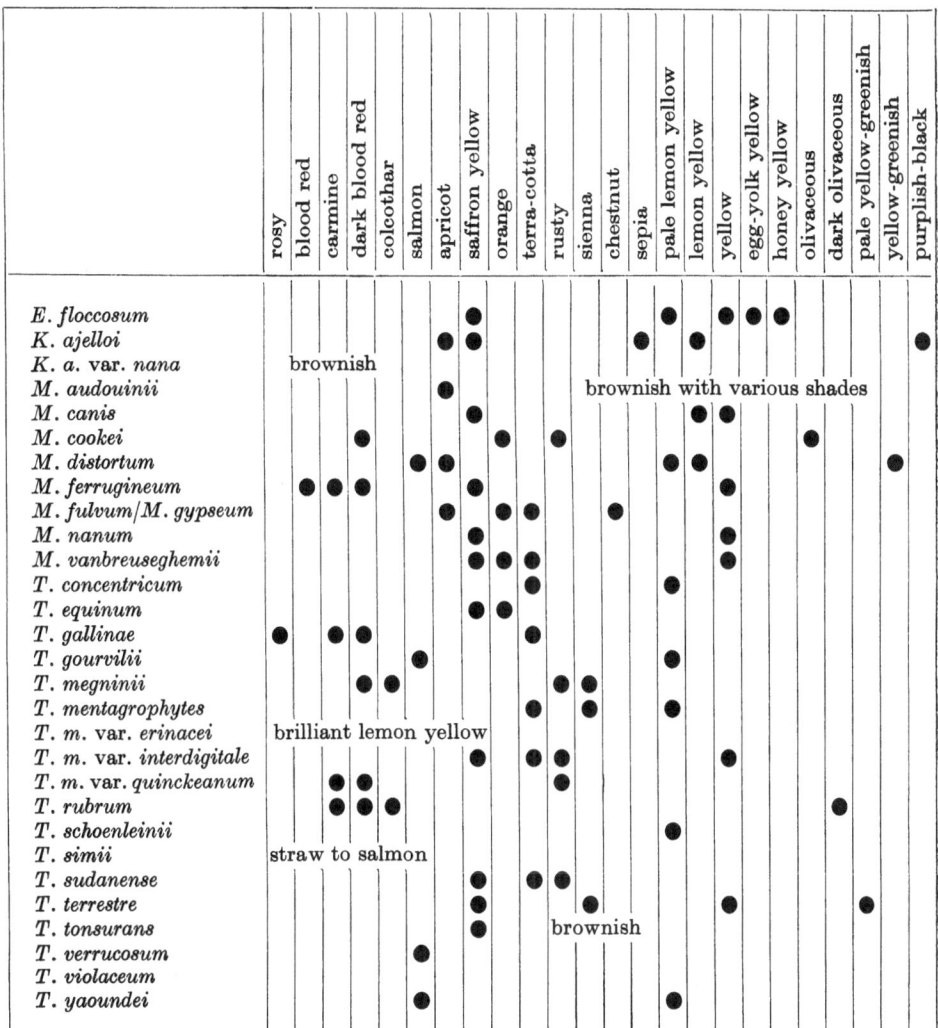

	rosy	blood red	carmine	dark blood red	coleothar	salmon	apricot	saffron yellow	orange	terra-cotta	rusty	sienna	chestnut	sepia	pale lemon yellow	lemon yellow	yellow	egg-yolk yellow	honey yellow	olivaceous	dark olivaceous	pale yellow-greenish	yellow-greenish	purplish-black
E. floccosum								•							•		•	•	•					
K. ajelloi							•	•								•	•							•
K. a. var. nana		brownish																						
M. audouinii							•						brownish with various shades											
M. canis								•								•	•							
M. cookei				•			•		•									•						
M. distortum						•	•	•								•	•						•	
M. ferrugineum		•	•	•				•									•							
M. fulvum/M. gypseum							•		•	•			•											
M. nanum								•	•	•							•							
M. vanbreuseghemii							•	•	•	•							•							
T. concentricum							•		•						•									
T. equinum								•	•															
T. gallinae	•		•	•					•															
T. gourvilii						•									•									
T. megninii			•	•							•	•												
T. mentagrophytes								•			•	•			•									
T. m. var. erinacei		brilliant lemon yellow																						
T. m. var. interdigitale								•	•	•							•							
T. m. var. quinckeanum			•	•						•														
T. rubrum			•	•	•																•			
T. schoenleinii															•									
T. simii		straw to salmon																						
T. sudanense								•	•	•														
T. terrestre								•	•				•				•					•		
T. tonsurans								•		brownish														
T. verrucosum						•																		
T. violaceum																								
T. yaoundei						•									•									

185

Table 13

The number of macroconidia

E. floccosum	numerous
K. ajelloi	numerous
K. a. var. *nana*	numerous
M. audouinii	mostly absent, sometimes in limited numbers
M. canis	numerous
M. cookei	numerous
M. distortum	numerous or in limited numbers
M. ferrugineum	not produced
M. fulvum/M. gypseum	numerous
M. nanum	numerous
M. vanbreuseghemii	numerous
T. concentricum	not produced
T. equinum	absent, in limited numbers, occ. numerous
T. gallinae	absent, in limited numbers, occ. numerous
T. gourvilii	absent, sometimes in limited numbers
T. megninii	absent, sometimes in limited numbers
T. mentagrophytes	in limited numbers or numerous
T. m. var. *erinacei*	numerous
T. m. var. *interdigitale*	not produced
T. m. var. *quinckeanum*	in limited numbers or numerous
T. rubrum	absent, in limited numbers, occ. numerous
T. schoenleinii	absent or few
T. simii	numerous
T. sudanense	not produced
T. terrestre	numerous
T. tonsurans	absent, in limited numbers, occ. numerous
T. verrucosum	absent or few
T. violaceum	absent or few
T. yaoundei	not produced

Table 14

The shapes of macroconidia

	egg-shaped	club-shaped	cylindrical	spindle-shaped	the wall*
E. floccosum	+	+	+		STn
K. ajelloi		+			} STk
K. a. var. nana	+				
M. audouinii				+	S/RTk
M. canis				+	
M. cookei				+	} RTk
M. distortum				+	
M. ferrugineum	not produced				
M. fulvum /M. gyp- seum				+	RTn
M. nanum	+				S/RTn
M. vanbreuseghemii			+	+	RTk
T. concentricum	not produced				
T. equinum		+			
T. gallinae		+	+	+	
T. gourvilii	irregular				} STn
T. megninii		+			
T. mentagrophytes		+			
T. m. var. erinacei	irregular				
T. m. var. inter- digitale	not produced				
T. m. var. quincke- anum		+		+	
T. rubrum		+	+		} STn
T. schoenleinii	irregular				
T. simii				+	
T. sudanense	not produced				
T. terrestre			+		
T. tonsurans		+			} STn
T. verrucosum	irregular				
T. violaceum	irregular				
T. yaoundei	not produced				

* S-smooth, R-rough, Tk-thick, Tn-thin

Table 15

The size of macroconidia

	Width × length in μm
E. floccosum	5—14 × 24—85 ·
K. ajelloi	8—19 × 16—40
K. a. var. nana	8—18 × 14—40
M. audouinii	8—25 × 30—190
M. canis	6—20 × 30—150
M. cookei	12—28 × 31—75
M. distortum	4—27 × 30—89
M. ferrugineum	not produced
M. fulvum/M. gypseum	6—18 × 24—80
M. nanum	4—12 × 11—24
M. vanbreuseghemii	8—13 × 44—88
T. concentricum	not produced
T. equinum	4—12 × 10—67
T. gallinae	5—10 × 15—56
T. gourvilii	4— 8 × 25—45
T. megninii	8—10 × 30—50
T. mentagrophytes	5—12 × 12—55
T. m. var. erinacei	irregular
T. m. var. interdigitale	not produced
T. m. var. quinckeanum	4—11 × 8—76
T. rubrum	4— 8 × 30—60
T. schoenleinii	4— 8 × 30—40
T. simii	6—11 × 35—85
T. sudanense	not produced
T. terrestre	3— 6 × 8—60
T. tonsurans	4—12 × 20—80
T. verrucosum	4— 8 × 16—50
T. violaceum	4— 6 × 30—40
T. yaoundei	not produced

Table 16

The number of microconidia

E. floccosum	absent
K. ajelloi	absent or found in limited numbers
K. a. var. *nana*	found in limited numbers
M. audouinii	absent or found in limited numbers
M. canis	
M. cookei	found in limited numbers
M. distortum	not too numerous or abundant
M. ferrugineum	absent
M. fulvum/M. gypseum	absent or found in limited numbers
M. nanum	
M. vanbreuseghemii	numerous
T. concentricum	absent
T. equinum	not too numerous or abundant
T. gallinae	absent or found in limited numbers
T. gourvilii	
T. megninii	
T. mentagrophytes	numerous
T. m. var. *erinacei*	
T. m. var. *interdigitale*	absent or found in limited numbers
T. m. var. *quinckeanum*	numerous
T. rubrum	absent or found in limited numbers
T. schoenleinii	absent
T. simii	found in limited numbers
T. sudanense	
T. terrestre	numerous
T. tonsurans	
T. verrucosum	absent or found in limited numbers
T. violaceum	
T. yaoundei	

189

Table 17

Experimental pathogenicity for guinea pig

	Pathogenic	Mostly weekly pathogenic or apathogenic
E. floccosum		+
K. ajelloi		+
K. a. var. *nana*		+
M. audouinii		+
M. canis	+	
M. cookei		+
M. distortum	+	
M. ferrugineum		+
M. fulvum/M. gypseum	+	
M. nanum	+	
M. vanbreuseghemii	+	
T. concentricum		+
T. equinum	+	
T. gallinae	+	
T. gourvilii	+	
T. megninii	+	
T. mentagrophytes	+	
T. m. var. *erinacei*	+	
T. m. var. *interdigitale*		+
T. m. var. *quinckeanum*	+	
T. rubrum		+
T. schoenleinii	+	
T. simii	+	
T. sudanense		+
T. terrestre		+
T. tonsurans	+	
T. verrucosum	+	
T. violaceum	+	
T. yaoundei		+

Table 18

The auxiliary identification of dermatophytes by hair keratinolysis of various animals and man

Dermatophyte \ Hair of	cattle	dog	goat	horse	mouse	man
E. floccosum	C + R	C	C	C + R	O	R
K. ajelloi	C + R	C	C	C	C	R
M. canis	C	C + R	C	C + R	C	R
M. gypseum	C	C + R	C	C	C	R
T. equinum	C	R	O	C + R	O	O
T. mentagrophytes	C	R	C	C	C	R
T. m. var. interdigitale	C	R	C	C	C	R
T. rubrum		C	C	C	C	C
T. terrestre	C + R	C + R	C	C	C	R
T. verrucosum	C	C	C	C	C	C

O — hair not attacked, C — coaxial, R — rectangular desintegration

191

Table 19

Nutritional tests

Dermatophyte	Casein	Casein-thiamine	Casein-inositol
T. concentricum	+	+	+
T. schoenleinii	+	+	+
T. verrucosum	0	$\pm^1$	x^2
T. mentagrophytes	+	+	
T. rubrum	+	+	
T. tonsurans	x	+	
M. ferrugineum	+	+	
T. violaceum	x	+	

Dermatophyte	Casein	Casein + Nicotinic acid
T. equinum	0	+
T. mentagrophytes	+	+

Dermatophyte	NH_4NO_3	NH_4NO_3 + histidine
T. megninii	0	+
T. gallinae	+	+

[1] most strains do not grow, some strains grow well, [2] the growth is poor

Table 20

The survey of perfect and corresponding imperfect states of dermatophytes

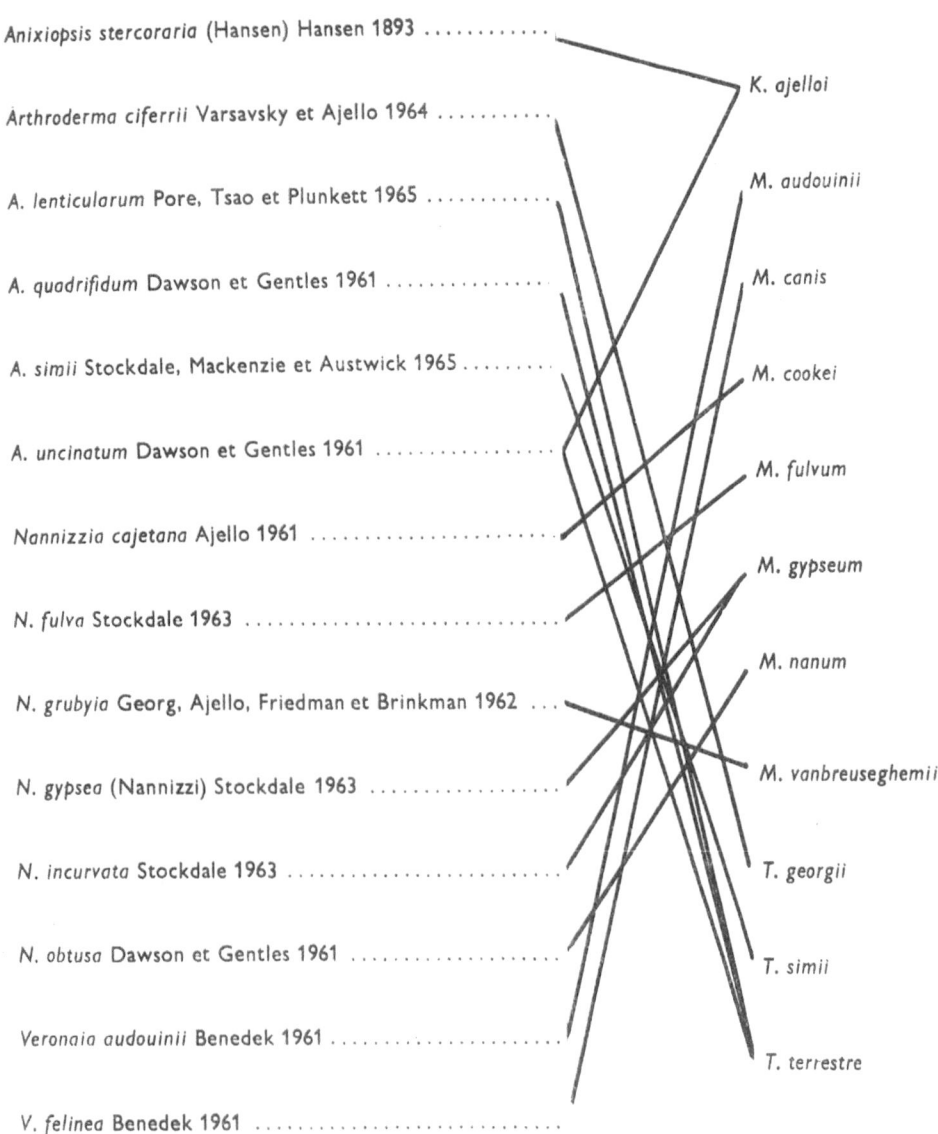

Anixiopsis stercoraria (Hansen) Hansen 1893 . . . .

Arthroderma ciferrii Varsavsky et Ajello 1964 . . . .

A. lenticularum Pore, Tsao et Plunkett 1965 . . . .

A. quadrifidum Dawson et Gentles 1961 . . . .

A. simii Stockdale, Mackenzie et Austwick 1965 . . . .

A. uncinatum Dawson et Gentles 1961 . . . .

Nannizzia cajetana Ajello 1961 . . . .

N. fulva Stockdale 1963 . . . .

N. grubyia Georg, Ajello, Friedman et Brinkman 1962 . . . .

N. gypsea (Nannizzi) Stockdale 1963 . . . .

N. incurvata Stockdale 1963 . . . .

N. obtusa Dawson et Gentles 1961 . . . .

Veronaia audouinii Benedek 1961 . . . .

V. felinea Benedek 1961 . . . .

K. ajelloi

M. audouinii

M. canis

M. cookei

M. fulvum

M. gypseum

M. nanum

M. vanbreuseghemii

T. georgii

T. simii

T. terrestre

Table 21

The survey of important signs of perfect states

Species	Size and colour of cleistothecia	Character of peridium	Peridial appendages	Imperfect states
A. lenticularum	300—600 µm pale yellow	terminal branches of hyphae usually with more than three cells, cells dumbbell-shaped, strongly constricted, mostly symmetrical	spirals of different length	T. terrestre
A. quadrifidum	400—700 µm light buff	cells of hyphae dumbbell-shaped, strongly constricted, asymmetrical. Their enlarged ends carry 1—2 protuberances on the turn of hypha	spirals of different length	
A. simii	200—750 µm light buff	terminal branches of hyphae with 2—3 cells at most, sometimes verticillate branching of hyphae, cells of inner peridial hyphae clavate, those of outer hyphae dumbbell-shaped, strongly constricted, mostly symmetrical	long spirals, with up to 20—30 turns	T. simii
A. uncinatum	300—900 µm buff	terminal branches of hyphae usually with more than three cells, cells dumbbell-shaped, strongly constricted, mostly symmetrical	spirals of different length	K. ajelloi
N. cajetana	400—700 µm light yellow	hyphae radial, often branched in verticillate manner, cells of hyphae cylindrical, without constriction	spirals of different length, tapered hyphae	M. cookei
N. fulva	500—1250 µm light buff	hyphae curved towards cleistothecium or radial side by side, otherwise as N. gypsea	spirals especially frequent, sometimes branched, tapered hyphae	M. fulvum
N. grubyia	150—600 µm light buff	hyphae curved towards cleistothecium, rarely branched in verticillate manner, cells of hyphae with single constriction in the middle	long spirals, with up to 30—50 turns, tapered hyphae	M. vanbreuseghemii

194

N. gypsea	300–750(900)μm light buff	hyphae curved towards cleistothecium, up to four branches in verticillate manner, cells of hyphae with 1—3 constrictions	spirals of different length, tapered hyphae	M. gypseum
N. incurvata	350–650(900)μm light buff	hyphae radial, often divided in up to five branches in verticillate manner, cells of hyphae with 1—3 constrictions	spirals of different length, tapered hyphae	
N. obtusa	250—450 μm buff	daughter and mother hyphae at one obtuse angle; they are curved over towards cleistothecium, verticillate branching is rare, cells with 1—2 constrictions	tight spirals, tapered hyphae	M. nanum

LITERATURE

AINSWORTH G. C. (1954): Fungoid infections of animals in Britain. Vet. Rec. 66, 1.

* AINSWORTH G. C. (1961): Ainsworth and Bisby's dictionary of the fungi. 5th ed., Commonw. Mycological Institute, Kew, Surrey.

AINSWORTH G. C., L. K. GEORG (1954): Nomenclature of the faviform Trichophytons. Mycologia 46, 9.

AINSWORTH G. C., P. K. C. AUSTWICK (1955): A survey of animal mycoses in Britain. General aspects. Vet. Rec. 67, 88.

* AINSWORTH G. C., P. K. C. AUSTWICK (1959): Fungal diseases of animals. Commonw. Agricult. Bur., Bucks.

AJELLO L. (1959): A new Microsporum and its occurrence in soil and on animals. Mycologia 51, 69.

AJELLO L. (1962): Present day concepts of the dermatophytes. Mycopath. Mycol. Appl. 17, 315.

* AJELLO L., L. K. GEORG, W. KAPLAN, L. KAUFMAN (1963): Laboratory manual for medical mycology. Public Health Service Publ., Washington.

ALTERAS I. (1965): Trichophyton quinckeanum infection in man. Brit. J. Derm. 77, 377.

ALTERAS I., M. CONU (1962): Un nouveau cas de dermatomycose humaine dû à T. gallinae. Considération sur la position de cette espèce dans la classification des dermatophytes. Mycopath. Mycol. Appl. 16, 247.

* ARIEVIČ A. M., Z. G. STĚPANIŠČEVA (1951): Atlas gribkovych zabolevanij koži. Medgiz, Moskva.

ASAJ A., M. HAJSIG, S. ČUTURIĆ (1965): Sanitary conditions in the management of calves and the occurrence of ringworm. Vet. Arch. 35, 1.

AUSTWICK P. K. C. (1966): Zoophilic dermatophytes as etiologic agents of ringworm in domestic animals. Abstracta III. Symp. Derm. Internat. Bratislava, 4.—6. 10., p. 17.

AZIMOV J. M. (1965): Někotorije voprosi epizootologii trichofytii krupnovo rogatovo skota v Azerbajdžanskoj SSR. Trudy Azerbajdž. nivn. 19, 13.

BALABANOFF V. A., L. B. KASAROV (1963): Production of macroconidia of Trichophyton megninii under the effect of carbon dioxide. Mycopath. Mycol. Appl. 19, 283.

BALABANOFF V. A., L. B. KASAROV (1963): Morphological changes of Trichophyton mentagrophytes under the influence of increased carbon dioxide tension. Mycopath. Mycol. Appl. 21, 161.

BALABANOFF V. A., L. B. KASAROV (1963): On the morphology of Trichophyton quinckeanum. Mycopath. Mycol. Appl. 21, 119.

---

* Textbooks and monographs.

BALABANOFF V. A., L. B. KASAROV (1963): Effects morphologiques du dioxyde de carbone sur les macroconidies de Keratinomyces ajelloi Vanbreuseghem. Ann. Parasit. hum. comp. 38, 131.

* BARNETT H. L. (1955): Illustrated genera of imperfect fungi. Burgess Publish. Co., Minneapolis, Minnesota.

BATTE E. G., W. S. MILLER (1963): Ringworm of horses and its control. J. Amer. vet. med. Ass. 123, 111.

BEARE M. J. (1958): Critical survey of mycological research and literature for the years 1946—1956 in Ireland. Mycopath. Mycol. Appl. 9, 65.

BEIRANA L., M. MAGANA (1960): Primer caso de tiña producido por Microsporum nanum en México. Bol. Derm. (Mexico) 1, 11.

BENEDEK T. (1961): Elicitation of perfect organ of fructification in Sabouraud's form-genus Microsporon (pro parte) by means of symbiosis with Bacillus weidmaniensis Benedek (1938). Mycopath. Mycol. Appl. 14, 101.

BENEDEK T. (1962): Fragmenta mycologica. II. On Castellani's "water cultures" and BENEDEK's "mycotheca" in chlorallactophenol. Mycopath. Mycol. Appl. 17, 255.

BENEDEK T. (1963): Fragmenta mycologica. IV. Use of thymol as an acaricidal agent against infestation of fungus cultures and mycotheca with acari (mites). Mycopath. Mycol. Appl. 19, 87.

BENEDEK T. (1963): On Anixiopsis stercoraria (Hansen) Hansen 1897 and its imperfect stage: Keratinomyces ajelloi Vanbreuseghem 1952. Mycopath. Mycol. Appl. 21, 179.

BENEDEK T. (1964): A new dermatophyte, Thallomicrosporon kuehnii Benedek 1963. Mycopath. Mycol. Appl. 23, 85.

BENEDEK T. (1964): Some remarks on cultures of dermatophytes on hair – on – soil medium. Mycopath. Mycol. Appl. 24, 331.

BENEDEK T. (1964): Hyphal fusion experiments between Microsporon gypseum (Bodin) Guiart and Grigoraki, 1928 and Keratinomyces ajelloi Vanbreuseghem, 1952. Riv. Pat. veget. III, 4, 411.

* BENEKE E. S. (1966): Medical mycology — laboratory manual. Burgess Publish. Co., Minneapolis, Minnesota.

BLAKEMORE J. C. (1965): Dermatophytosis (ringworm): Pathogenesis, diagnosis and treatment. J. Amer. vet. med. Ass. 147, 1470.

BLANK F., L. P. EREAUX (1964): Die Dermatophytenflora der Provinz Quebec. Hautarzt 15, 670.

BORELLI D. (1965): Microsporum racemosum, nova species. Acta med. Venezol. 12, 148.

BROCK J. M. (1961): Microsporum nanum. A cause of tinea capitis. A case report. Arch. Derm. (Chicago) 84, 504.

BROOKS B. E., H. A. JOSEPH, C. C. CAMPBELL (1959): Isolation of Microsporum distortum from a human case. J. invest. Derm. 33, 23.

BROWN G. W., G. F. DONALD (1964): Equine ringworm due to Trichophyton mentagrophytes var. quinckeanum. Mycopath. Mycol. Appl. 23, 269.

BUBASH G. R., O. J. GINTHER, L. AJELLO (1964): Microsporum nanum: First recorded isolation from animals in the United States. Science 143, 366.

BUCHVALD J. (1964): Prvá epizoócia trichofýcie u koní na Slovensku, vyvolaná Trichophyton equinum. Čs. epid. mikrob. imunol. 13, 286.

BUCHWALD J. (1965): Historický prehlad rozvoja dermatomykológie na Slovensku s prihliadnutím k epidemiologickej situácii výskytu dermatomykóz na slovenskom území. Čs. derm. 40, 65.

BUCHWALD J. (1965): Príspevok k problematike živočišnych rezervoárov trichofýcie a hodnotenie ich významu pre človeka. Čs. epid. mikrob. imunol. 14, 289.

BUCHWALD J., M. VALENTOVÁ (1965): Vzácný výskyt trichofytickej nákazy človeka zapríčinený Trichophyton equinum (Matruchot et Dassonville 1898, Gedoelst 1902). Čs. derm. 40, 115.

BÜHLMANN X., H. RIETH (1962): Über die Erkennung und Bedeutung von Dermatomykosen bei Haustieren. Schweiz. Arch. Tierheilk. 104, 537.

CARMICHAEL J. W., J. F. REID (1961): Microsporum nanum infection in Alberta. Mycopath. Mycol. Appl. 17, 49.

CARNAGHAN R. B. A., M. GITTER, J. D. BLAXLAND (1956): Favus in poultry: an outbreak of Trichophyton gallinae infection. Vet. Rec. 68, 600.

CARTER G. R., M. V. GLENN (1966): Ringworm with complicating acanthosis in swine. J. Amer. vet. med. Ass. 149, 42.

CASTELLANI A. (1960): A brief note on the viability of some pathogenic fungi in sterile distilled water and a simple method to maintain fungal strains in mycological collections, preventing pleomorphism. Imprensa Méd. 24, 270.

CASTELLANI A. (1963): The "water cultivation" of pathogenic fungi. J. trop. Med. Hyg. 66, 283.

CETIN E. T., M. TAHSINOGLU, S. VOLKAN (1965): Epizootic of Trichophyton mentagrophytes (interdigitale) in white mice. Path. Microbiol. 28, 839.

CHIN B., S. G. KNIGHT (1957): Growth of Trichophyton mentagrophytes and Trichophyton rubrum in increased carbon dioxide tensions. J. gen. Microbiol. 16, 642.

CHMEL L. (1946): Výskyt dermatofytov na Slovensku v období 1942—1946. Brat. lék. listy 26, 1.

* CHMEL L. (1964): Štúdia o epidemiológii a experimentálnej terapii dermatomykóz. Vydavatelstvo SAV, Bratislava.

* CONANT N. F., D. T. SMITH, R. D. BAKER, J. L. CALLAWAY, D. S. MARTIN (1964): Manual of clinical mycology. 2nd ed. Saunders, Philadelphia, London.

CONNOLE M. D. (1963): A review of dermatomycoses of animals in Australia. Aust. vet. J. 39, 130.

CONNOLE M. D. (1965): Keratinophilic fungi on cats and dogs. Sabouraudia 4, 45.

CONNOLE M. D., J. D. BAYNES (1966): Ringworm caused by Microsporum nanum in pigs. Aust. vet. J. 42, 19.

CONROY J. D. (1964): Microsporum infections in cats. J. Amer. vet. med. Ass. 145, 115.

* COUDERT J. (1955): Guide pratique de mycologie médical. Masson et Cie édit., Paris.

COUDERT J. (1964): Répartition géographique des dermatophytes en Europe. Ann. Soc. belge Méd. trop. 44, 725.

COUDERT M., M. R. BATTESTI, J. MICHEL-BRUN (1966): Evolution du concept de dermatophyte. Lyon méd. 18, 1217.

ČUTURIĆ S., S. RICHTER (1965): Pojava trichofitije u jednom uzgoju kokoši. Vet. Arch. 35, 256.

* DALLDORF G. (1962): Fungi and fungous diseases. Charles C. Thomas, Springfield, Ill.

DAVIDSON A. M., E. S. DOWDING, H. R. BULLER (1932): Hyphal fusion in dermatophytes. Canad. J. Res. 6, 1.

DAWSON C. O., J. C. GENTLES (1961): The perfect states of Keratinomyces ajelloi Vanbreuseghem, Trichophyton terrestre Durie et Frey and Microsporum nanum Fuentes. Sabouraudia 1, 49.

DAWSON C. O., J. C. GENTLES, E. M. BROWN (1964): Environmental conditions affecting sexual reproduction in species of Arthroderma and Nannizzia. Sabouraudia 3, 245.

De Keyser J., L. Delcambe, D. Thienpont (1960): Activité thérapeutique de l'iturine et du chinosol sur la teigne du cheval à Microsporum equinum Bodin. Bull. épizoot. Dis. Afrique 8, 279.

De Keyser J., Cotteleer (1961): Haaruitval bij twee chinchilla's veroorzaakt door Ctenomyces mentagrophytes (Robin-Blanchard). Vlaams Diergeneesk. T. 30, 177.

Di Menna M., M. J. Marples (1954): Microsporum distortum sp. nov. from New Zealand. Trans. Brit. Mycol. Soc. 37, 372.

* Dočekal B., J. Dvořák (1954): Příručka lékařské mykologie. Státní zdravot. naklad. Praha.

Dodd D. C., R. W. Newlin, G. R. Niksch (1965): Infection of swine with Microsporum nanum. J. Amer. vet. med. Ass. 146, 486.

* Dodge C. W. (1935): Medical mycology. C. V. Mosby Co., St. Louis.

Donald G. F., G. Brown (1964): T. mentagrophytes and T. mentagrophytes var. quinckeanum infections of South Australian mice. Aust. J. Derm. 7, 133.

* Dubos R. J., J. G. Hirsch (1965): Bacterial and mycotic infections of man. Lippincott Co., Philadelphia.

Dvořák J. (1957): Die Anastomosierungsfähigkeit heterogener Dermatophytenhyphen. Zbl. Bakt. II. Orig. 110, 697.

Dvořák J., Přikryl, J. Sobota (1959): Pokusy o izolaci dermatofytů z půdy. Čs. epid. mikrob. imunol. 4, 259.

Dvořák J., M. Otčenášek (1964): The isolation of Trichophyton gallinae (Mégnin) Silva et Benham 1952 from man. J. invest. Derm. 42, 3.

Dvořák J., M. Otčenášek (1964): Geophilic, zoophilic and anthropophilic dermatophytes. Mycopath. Mycol. Appl. 23, 294.

Dvořák J., M. Otčenášek (1965): Die Änderungen der relativen Frequenzen der Dermatophytosenerreger bei ostböhmischen Patienten im letzten Dezennium. Hautarzt 16, 353.

Dvořák J., M. Otčenášek, J. Komárek (1965): Das Spektrum der aus Tierläsionen in Ostböhmen in den Jahren 1962—1964 isolierten Dermatophyten. Mykosen 8, 126.

Dvořák J., M. Otčenášek, G. Silva Taboada (1965): Informe preliminar sobre el estudio dermatofitológico de los suelos de La Habana. Poeyana (Habana) Ser. A, 8, 1.

Dvořák J., M. Otčenášek (1966): Ein Beitrag zu den sog. dermatophytischen Mischkulturen. Mykosen 9, 161.

Dvořák J., M. Otčenášek (1967): Einige Bemerkungen zur Systematik der Dermatophyten. Mykosen 10,571.

Dvořák J., Z. Hubálek, M. Otčenášek (1968): The "in vitro" survival of dermatophytes in human skin scales. Arch. Derm. 98,540.

Dvořák J., Z. Hubálek, M. Otčenášek (1969): The influence of some preparatory fluids on the morphology of adiaspores and macroconidia. Folia parasitologica — in press.

Ek N. (1965): Von durch T. verrucosum var. discoides verursachte Glatzflechte bei Ferkeln. Nord. Vet.-Med. 17, 152.

El Fiki A. Y. (1959): Inaugural dissertation. Tierärztl. Hochschule, Hannover.

* Emmons C. W., C. H. Binford, J. P. Utz (1963): Medical mycology. Lea and Febiger, Philadelphia.

English M. P. (1961): An outbreak of equine ringworm due to Trichophyton equinum. Vet. Rec. 73, 578.

English M. P. (1964): The ecology of some keratinophilic fungi associated with hedgehogs. N. Z. med. J. 63, 586.

ENGLISH M. P., J. M. B. SMITH, F. M. RUSH-MUNRO (1964): Hedgehog ringworm in the North Island of New Zealand. N. Z. med. J. 63, 40.

EVOLCEANU R., I. ALTERAS, I. COJOCARU (1964): Dermatomycoses provoquées par les dermatophytes d'origine tellurique. Ann. Derm. Syph. (Paris) 91, 127.

FLÓRIÁN E., L. FARKAS (1958): Eine durch Trichophyton (Achorion) gallinae verursachte Kopfmykose. Börgyógy. vener. Szle 12, 85.

FLÓRIÁN E., J. GALGÓCZY (1964): Keratinomyces longifusus sp. nov. from Hungary. Mycopath. Mycol. Appl. 24, 73.

FLÓRIÁN E., J. GALGÓCZY, E. K. NOVÁK (1964): Are Microsporon distortum di Menna et Marples 1954 and Microsporon umbonatum Sabouraud 1907 identical? Mycopath. Mycol. Appl. 23, 39.

* FRÁGNER P. (1958): Parasitische Pilze beim Menschen. Nakladatelství ČSAV, Praha.

FRÁGNER P. (1964): Vlastní zkušenosti s cycloheximidem, chloramfenikolem a desertomycinem v selektivních půdách pro mykologickou kultivaci. Čs. epid. mikrob. imunol. 13, 48.

FREY D., E. B. DURIE, R. F. A. BECKE (1960): Isolation of Microsporum distortum from two children with ringworm of the scalp. Aust. J. Derm. 5, 1.

FRIEDRICH E. (1964): Perforation von Frauenhaar durch Dermatophyten I. Z. Haut.-Geschl. Krkh. 36, 39.

FRIEDRICH E. (1964): Perforation von Frauenhaar durch Dermatophyten II. Mykosen 7, 53.

FUENTES C. A. (1956): A new species of Microsporum. Mycologia 48, 613.

FUENTES C. A., R. ABOULAFIA, R. J. VIDAL (1954): A dwarf form of Microsporum gypseum. J. invest. Derm. 23, 51.

GEMEINHARDT H. (1965): Zur Frage der selektiven Anzüchtung von Dermatophyten durch Desertomycin. Derm. Wschr. 151, 756.

GENTLES J. C., J. G. O'SULLIVAN (1957): Correlation of human and animal ringworm in west of Scotland. Brit. med. J. 21, 678.

GENTLES J. C., C. O. DAWSON, M. D. CONNOLE (1965): Keratinophilic fungi on cats and dogs. Sabouraudia 4, 171.

GEORG L. K. (1960): Epidemiology of the dermatophytoses sources of infection, modes of transmission and epidemicity. Ann. N. Y. Acad. Sci 89, 69.

GEORG L. K. (1964): Ecology and diagnostic problems of fungal zoonoses. Industr. Med. Surg. 33, 308.

GEORG L. K., E. H. MAECHLING (1949): Trichophyton mentagrophytes (variety nodular). A mutant with brilliant orange red pigment isolated in nine cases of ringworm of the skin and nails. J. invest. Derm. 13, 339.

GEORG L. K., W. KAPLAN, L. B. CAMP (1957): Trichophyton equinum — a re-evaluation of its taxonomic status. J. invest. Derm. 29, 27.

GEORG L. K., W. KAPLAN, B. C. LA VERNE (1957): Equine ringworm with special reference to Trichophyton equinum. Amer. J. vet. Res. 18, 798.

GEORG L. K., W. KAPLAN, L. AJELLO, W. M. WILLIAMSON, E. B. TILDEN (1959): The parasitic nature of the soil fungus Keratinomyces ajelloi. J. invest. Derm. 32, 539.

GEORG L. K., L. AJELLO, L. FRIEDMAN, S. A. BRINKMAN (1962): A new species of Microsporum pathogenic to man and animals. Sabouraudia 1, 189.

GEORG L. K., L. AJELLO, A. NOVICK, E. R. PRICE, A. E. BLUM (1963): Ringworm due to M. vanbreuseghemii in a dog. J. Amer. vet. med. Ass. 143, 596.

GEORG L. K., P. DOUPAGNE, S. R. PATTYN, H. NEVES (1963): Trichophyton yaoundei: a dermatophyte indigenous to Africa. J. invest. Derm. 41, 19.

Gierloff B. C. H., J. Katič (1961): Om anvendelse af griseofulvin specielt i veterinaer praksis. Nord. Vet.-Med. 13, 571.

Ginther O. J. (1965): Clinical aspects of Microsporum nanum infection in swine. J. Amer. vet. med. Ass. 146, 945.

Ginther O. J., L. Ajello, G. R. Bubash, E. Varsavsky (1964): First American isolations of Trichophyton mentagrophytes in swine. Vet. Med. 59, 1038.

Ginther O. J., G. R. Bubash, L. Ajello (1964): Microsporum nanum infection in swine. Vet. Med. 59, 79.

Ginther O. J., G. R. Bubash, L. Ajello, P. E. Fenwick (1964): Microsporum nanum infection in swine in four states. Vet. Med. 59, 490.

Gip L. (1964): Isolation of Trichophyton gallinae from two patients with tinea cruris. Acta derm.-venereol. (Stock.) 44, 251.

Gip L., B. O. Martin (1964): Isolation of Trichophyton terrestre, Trichophyton mentagrophytes var. asteroides and Trichophyton rubrum from dogs. Acta derm.-venereol. (Stock.) 44, 248.

* Götz H. (1962): Die Pilzkrankheiten der Haut durch Dermatophyten. Bd. IV/3. Springer Verl., Berlin, Göttingen, Heidelberg.

Götz H. (1964): Remarks on the classification of dermatophytes. Ann. Soc. belge Méd. trop. 44, 693.

Grin E. I., L. Ožegović (1959): Problemi attuali delle dermatomicosi in Iugoslavia. Minerva med. 50, 1245.

Gründer H. D. (1965): Beitrag zur Bekämpfung der Trichophytie beim Rind. Berl. Münch. tierärztl. Wschr. 78, 261.

Hajsig M., M. Žuković (1961): Isolacija Trichophyton verrucosum s usi i pauci goveda i istrazivanji utjecaja desinfektiji na tok trichofitija. Vet. Arch. 31, 225.

Hauser W., Heymer (1964): Beobachtung von T. sudanense in Deutschland. Z. Haut-Geschl. Krkh. 37, 106.

* Hazen E. L., F. C. Reed (1960): Laboratory identification of pathogenic fungi simplified. 2nd ed., Charles C. Thomas, Springfield, Ill.

Hejtmánek M. (1957): O variabilitě šesti kmeňů Trichophyton ferrugineum (Ota 1921) Langeron et Milochevitch 1930 a specifitě vegetativních anastomos mezi nimi. Scripta med. 30, 319.

Hejtmánek M. (1959): K vegetativním anastomosám mezi hyfami dermatofytů. Acta univ. Palack. olomuc. 18, 21.

Hejtmánek M. (1959): Saprofytická stádia dermatofytů v přírodě. Biológia (Bratislava) 12, 928.

Hejtmánek M. (1962): První izolace Microsporum cookei Ajello 1959 na území ČSSR. Čs. epid. mikrob. imunol. 11, 127.

Hejtmánek M. (1964): Zum Problem des Pleomorphismus — morphophysiologische und genetische Aspekte. Ann. Soc. belge Méd. trop. 44, 852.

Hejtmánek M. (1966): O soudobé koncepci klasifikace a nomenklatury v dermatomykologii. Čs. derm. 41, 126.

Hejtmánek M. (1967): Private communication.

Hejtmánková-Uhrová N. (1966): Über eine Methode der Mikrokultivierung der perfekten Stadien und die Ascosporenfärbung bei Microsporon gypseum (Bodin) Guiart et Grigoraki. Mycopath. Mycol. Appl. 29, 182.

Hilbrich P. (1958): Das Huhn — ein wirtschaftlicher Faktor. Farbenfabrik Bayer A. G., Hannover.

* Hübschmann K., P. Frágner (1962): Dermatofyta a kožní choroby jimi vyvolané. Nakladatelství ČSAV, Praha.

JAKSCH W. (1963): Dermatomykosen der Equiden, Karnivoren und einiger Rodentien in Österreich, mit einem Beitrag zur normalen Pilzflora der Haut. Wien. tierärztl. Mschr. 50, 831.

JAKSCH W. (1963): Dermatomykosen der Equiden, Karnivoren und einiger Rodentien in Österreich, mit einem Beitrag zur normalen Pilzflora der Haut. Wien. tierärztl. Mschr. 50, 904.

JAKSCH W. (1963): Dermatomykosen der Equiden, Karnivoren und einiger Rodentien in Österreich, mit einem Beitrag zur normalen Pilzflora der Haut. Wien. tierärztl. Mschr. 50, 1076.

JAKSCH W. (1965): Mykosen der Tiere als Infektionsquelle des Menschen. Wien. tierärztl. Mschr. 52, 723.

JAKSCH W., J. THURNER (1966): Private communication.

JUNGERMAN P. J. (1965): Diagnosis and treatment of animal mycoses. Sthwest. Vet. 18, 2.

KABEN U. (1964): Erstmalige Isolierung von Trichophyton soudanense Joyeux in Deutschland. Mykosen 7, 82.

KABEN U. (1964): Über die Isolierung eines atypischen Microsporum canis-Stammes von einem Weisshandgibbon (Hylobates lar). Mykosen 7, 115.

KABEN U., W. D. PLÖTZ (1962): Mäusefavus im Bereich des behaarten Kopfes. Derm. Wschr. 146, 270.

KAMYSZEK F. (1966): Dermatomykozy zwierzat jako zródlo zarazenia ludzi. Med. weteryn. 22, 90.

KAPLAN W., L. K. GEORG, S. L. HENDRIKS, R. A. LEEPER (1957): Isolation of Microsporum distortum from animals in the United States. J. invest. Derm. 28, 449.

* KAŠKIN P. N. (1962): Medicinskaja mikologia. Medgiz, Leningrad.

KEEP J. M. (1959): The epidemiology of Microsporum canis (Bodin) in a cat community. Aust. vet. J. 35, 374.

KEEP J. M. (1963): A survey of Microsporum canis infection of cats in Sydney. Aust. vet. J. 39, 330.

KIELSTEIN P. (1963): Zur Anwendung verschiedener Pilzhemmungsmittel für die selektive kulturelle Isolierung von Trichophytonarten. Mh. Vet.-Med. 18, 111.

KIELSTEIN P. (1964): Zur Epidemiologie und Pathogenese der Trichophytie unter besonderer Berücksichtigung der veterinär- und humanmedizinischen Literatur. Mh. Vet.-Med. 19, 174.

KIELSTEIN P. (1965): Untersuchungen zur Pathogenese der Rindertrichophytie I. Arch. exp. Vet. Med. 19, 629.

KIELSTEIN P. (1965): Untersuchungen zur Pathogenese der Rindertrichophytie II. Arch. exp. Vet. Med. 19, 885.

KIELSTEIN P., E. RÖHR (1962): Probleme der Epidemiologie und mykologischen Diagnose der Rindertrichophytie. Arch. exp. Vet. Med. 16, 477.

KIELSTEIN P., W. WELLER (1965): Trichophyton verrucosum-Infektionen bei Schafen. Mh. Vet.-Med. 20, 671.

KIELSTEIN P., V. A. BALABANOFF (1966): Trichophyton verrucosum Bodin (1902) — a highly differentiated zoophilous dermatophyte. Mh. Vet.-Med. 21, 16.

KLOKKE A. H., G. A. DE VRIES (1963): Tinea capitis in chimpanzees caused by Microsporum canis Bodin 1902 resembling M. obesum Conant 1937. Sabouraudia 2, 268.

KOMINAMI M. (1960): A survey of keratinolytic or keratinophilic molds from soil in Japan. III. The identification of Trichophyton lipoferum sp. nov. Shinkin to Shinkinsho 2, 38.

KRAL F. (1955): Classification, symptomatology and recent treatment of animal dermatomycoses (ringworm). J. Amer. vet. med. Ass. 127, 395.

KRAL F. (1960): Skin infection in animals. Vet. Med. 55, 48.

* KRAL F. (1960): Compendium of veterinary dermatology. Pfizer, New York.

KRAL F. (1962): Skin diseases. Advanc. vet. Sci. 7, 183.

KRAL F. (1963): Mykosen der Hunde und Katzen. Berl. Münch. tierärztl. Wschr. 76, 333.

* KRAL F. (1964): Veterinary dermatology. Lippincott Co., Philadelphia.

* KRAL F., R. M. SCHWARTZMANN (1964): Veterinary and comparative dermatology. Lippincott Co., Philadelphia and Montreal.

KRENTEL G., K. KÜHNE (1962): Vorläufige Mitteilung über Untersuchungergebnisse bei menschlichen Trichophytien und Rindertrichophytien in der Umgebung von Magdeburg. Mykosen 5, 122.

KUNERT J., M. HEJTMÁNEK (1964): Izolace nového dermatofyta rodu Keratinomyces Vanbreuseghem 1952. Čs. epid. mikrob. imunol. 13, 293.

KUNERT J., M. OTČENÁŠEK (1968): Perfect states of dermatophytes. Čes. mykologie 22,56.

LANGER J. (1953): Microsporon ferrugineum, jeho první izolace na území naší republiky. Čs. derm. 28, 446.

LANGER J., H. BÖHME (1965): Zur Epidemiologie und Pathogenese der Trichophytie unter besonderer Berücksichtigung der veterinär- und humanmedizinischen Literatur. Mykosen 8, 1.

* LANGERON M., R. VANBREUSEGHEM (1952): Précis de mycologie. Masson et Cie édit., Paris.

LA TOUCHE C. J. (1960): Mouse favus due to Trichophyton quinckeanum (Zopf) Mac Leod et Muende: a reappraisal in the light of recent investigations. IV. Mycopath. Mycol. Appl. 13, 33.

LA TOUCHE C. J., R. A. FORSTER (1963): Spontaneous infection in the hedgehog (Erinaceus europaeus) by a variety of Trichophyton mentagrophytes (Robin) Blanchard. Sabouraudia 2, 143.

LENHART K., M. HEJTMÁNEK (1963): O závislosti tvaru makrokonidií na stáří kolonie. Acta univ. Palack. olomuc. 33, 237.

* LEWIS G. M., M. E. HOOPER, J. W. WILSON, O. A. PLUNKETT (1958): An introduction to medical mycology. 4th ed., Year Book Publish., Inc., Chicago, Ill.

LONDERO A. T., O. FISCHMAN, C. D. RAMOS (1963): An epizootic of Trichophyton equinum infection on horses in Brasil. Sabouraudia 3, 14.

LONDERO A. T., O. FISCHMAN, C. D. RAMOS (1964): Trichophyton gallinae in Brasil. Sabouraudia 3, 233.

MACKENZIE D. W. R. (1963): "Hairbrush diagnosis" in detection and eradication of non-fluorescent scalp ringworm. Brit. med. J. 2, 363.

MAKMINYA E. M. (1963): Ringworm in nutrias. Krolikov. zverev. 6, 25.

MANYCH J., J. KEJDA (1966): Nález neobvyklého druhu dermatofyta v onychomykotické lézi. Čs. epid. mikrob. imunol. 15, 62.

MARAIS V., D. L. OLIVIER (1965): Isolation of Trichophyton mentagrophytes from a porcupine. Sabouraudia 4, 49.

MARIAT F., G. TAPIA (1966): Observations sur une souche de Microsporum cookei parasite du cynocephale (Papio papio). Sabouraudia 5, 43.

MARPLES M. J., J. M. B. SMITH (1960): The hedgehog as a source of human ringworm. Nature (Lond.) 188, 867.

McGABE M. G., P. D. MIER (1960): Pigments of trichophyta. J. gen. Microbiol. 23, 1.

* MOSS E. S., A. L. McQUOWN (1960): Atlas of medical mycology. Williams-Wilkins Co., Baltimore.

Novák E., J. Galgóczy (1963): A dermatophyton gombák perfekt alakja és renszertani helysete. Börgyógy. vener. Szle 39, 1.

Obrtel J. (1936): Morfologické a biologické vlastnosti kožních plísní v Praze se vyskytujících. Čs. derm. 16, 1.

* Obrtel J. (1950): Dermatophyta. Stát. zdrav. naklad. Praha.

Okoshi S., M. Takashio (1963): A case of equine ringworm caused by Microsporum gypseum. Jap. J. Vet. Sci. 25, 203.

Okoshi S., A. Hasegawa (1964): Canine and feline ringworm caused by Microsporum canis. Jap. J. Vet. Sci. 26, 57.

Otčenášek M., J. Dvořák (1962): The isolation of Trichophyton terrestre and other keratinophilic fungi from small mammals of South Eastern Moravia. Sabouraudia 2, 111.

Otčenášek M., J. Dvořák, Z. Sova (1962): Das gehäufte Auftreten einer Dermatophytose bei der Grosszucht von Pferden. Mykosen 5, 131.

Otčenášek M., J. Dvořák, J. Komárek (1964): K mykologické diagnostice trichofýcií vyvolávaných Trichophyton verrucosum Bodin 1902. Vet. Med. (Praha) 9, 391.

Otčenášek M., J. Dvořák, M. Šabatová, E. Horáková (1964): Zwei Befunde der Trichophyton equinum (Matruchot et Dassonville) Gedoelst 1902 in menschlichen Läsionen. Derm. Wschr. 149, 438.

Otčenášek M., J. Dvořák, G. Silva Taboada (1965): Dermatofitos y otros hongos queratinofílicos en los suelos de Cuba. Poeyana (Habana) Sr. A, 13, 1.

Otčenášek M., J. Dvořák, K. Ladzianska (1967): Trichophyton rubrum-like dermatophyte as a causative agent of dermatophytosis in chimpanzees. Mycopath. Mycol. Appl. 31, 33.

Ožegović L. (1957): Dermatophytes and their treatment in veterinary text books. Veterinaria (Sarajevo) 6, 1.

Ožegović L. (1964): Erfahrungen mit der Rindertrichophytie in Jugoslawien. Dtsch. tierärztl. Wschr. 71, 34.

Ožegović L., R. Pavlović (1961): Trichophytosis in cattle at agricultural estates — disease of the herd. Veterinaria (Sarajevo) 10, 57.

Ožegović L., E. I. Grin (1963): Epidemiologische Bedeutung der animalen Dermatophytien in Jugoslawien. Wien. tierärztl. Mschr. 50, 1037.

* Paclt J. (1958): Farbenbestimmung in der Biologie. VEB Gustav Fischer Verl., Jena.

Paldrok H. (1953): On the variability and classification of dermatophytes. Acta derm.-venereol. (Stockh.) 33, 1.

Partridge B. M. (1959): Hair penetration by dermatophytes with special reference to its use in the diagnosis of Trichophyton rubrum. Trans. St. John's Hosp. Derm. Soc. (Lond.) 42, 52.

Pätiälä R. (1951): On fungus diseases in game. Papers Gam. Res. 6, 21.

Petzold K., K. H. Böhm (1965): Untersuchungen über den Befall von Raubkatzen mit Microsporum canis. Dtsch. tierärztl. Wschr. 72, 461.

Petzold K., H. Rieth, H. Merkt (1965): Enzootien durch Trichophyton equinum bei Pferden. Dtsch. tierärztl. Wschr. 72, 302.

Pier A. C., I. P. Hughes (1961): Isolation of Keratinomyces ajelloi from skin lesions of a horse. J. Amer. vet. med. Ass. 138, 484.

Quaife R. A. (1966): Human infection due to the hedgehog fungus, Trichophyton mentagrophytes var. erinacei. J. clin. Path. 19, 177.

Rdzanek I., D. Weyman-Rzucidlo, Z. Pohorecka (1963): Infection due to Trichophyton quinckeanum (Mouse favus). Przegl. derm. 50, 272.

* Rebell G., D. Taplin, H. Blank (1964): Dermatophytes. Their recognition and identification. Dermatology Foundation of Miami.

Refai M. (1966): Ringworm in buffalos caused by Trichophyton violaceum in Egypt. Abstracta III. Symp. Derm. Internat. Bratislava 4.—6. 10., p. 22.

Refai M., H. Rieth, K. Ito (1964): Zur Identifizierung von Trichophyton mentagrophytes und Trichophyton rubrum auf Glukose und Peptonlösung. Bull. Pharm. Res. Inst. 54, 1.

Rieth H. (1958): Mykosen bei Tieren. Ther. Berichte 30, 151.

Rieth H., A. Y. El-Fiki (1958): Renaissance der animalen Mykologie. Berl. Münch. tierärztl. Wschr. 71, 391.

Rioux J. A., D. T. Jarry, B. Juminer (1964): Un nouveau dermatophyte isolé du sol: Trichophyton vanbreuseghemii n. sp. Naturalia Monspel. Ser. Bot. 16, 153.

Rippon J. W., M. Medenica (1964): Isolation of Trichophyton soudanense in the United States. Sabouraudia 3, 301.

Rittenbach P., H. Günther (1963): Beiträge zur Pathologie tierischer Mykosen. Mh. Vet.-Med. 18, 887.

Rivalier E. (1954): Description de Sabouraudites praecox nova species suivie de remarques sur le genre Sabouraudites. Ann. Inst. Pasteur 86, 276.

Rosetti N. (1942): Achorion gallinae (Mégnin-Sabrazès, 1890—93). Caso de infestação humana expontânea. Rev. Inst. A. Lutz (S. Paolo) 2, 288.

* Sabouraud R. (1910): Maladies du cuir chevelu. III. Les maladies cryptogamiques. Les Teignes. Masson et Cie édit., Paris.

Sarkany I., G. Midley (1966): Trichophyton yaoundei infection in Britain. Brit. J. Derm. 78, 225.

Schönborn Ch. (1966): Untersuchungen über die Vitalität von Dermatophyten im Erdboden. Arch. klin. exp. Derm. 224, 268.

Schönborn Ch. (1966): Trichophyton soudanense (Joyeux 1912) als Erreger einer Fuss- und Nagelmykose. Derm. Wschr. 152, 5.

Seeliger H. P. R., W. Bisping, H. P. Brandt (1963): Über eine Microsporum-Enzootie bei Kappen-Gibbons (Hylobates lar) verursacht durch eine Variante von Microsporum canis. Mykosen 6, 61.

* Segretain G., E. Drouhet, F. Mariat (1964): Le diagnostic de laboratoire en mycologie médicale. 2e édit. La Tourelle.

Silva M., R. W. Benham (1952): Nutritional studies of the dermatophytes with special reference to Trichophyton megninii Blanchard 1896 and Trichophyton gallinae (Megnin 1881) comb. nov. J. invest. Derm. 18, 453.

* Simons R. D. (1954): Medical mycology. Cleaver-Hume Press Ltd., London.

Smith J. M. B., M. J. Marples (1963): Trichophyton mentagrophytes var. erinacei. Sabouraudia 3, 1.

* Spesivtseva N. A. (1964): Mikozy i mokotoksikozy životnych. Gos. Izd. Sel-choz. lit. Moskva.

Stockdale P. M. (1963): The Microsporum gypseum complex (Nannizzia incurvata Stock., N. gypsea (Nann.) comb. nov., N. fulva sp. nov.). Sabouraudia 3, 114.

Stockdale P. M., D. W. R. Mackenzie, P. K. C. Austwick (1965): Arthroderma simii sp. nov., the perfect state of Trichophyton simii (Pinoy) comb. nov. Sabouraudia 4, 112.

Šik G. (1965): Microsporia on the smooth skin, caused by Microsporum cookei Ajello 1959. Derm. Vener. (Sofia) 4, 6.

Taylor W. W., F. Radcliffe, P. F. D. Van Peenen (1964): A survey of small Egyptian mammals for pathogenic fungi. Sabouraudia 3, 140.

THURNER J. (1966): Studien über das keratinolytische Vermögen der Dermatophyten. I. Mitteilung. Keratinabbau durch Dermatophyten an verschiedenen Haaren. Arch. klin. exp. Derm. 224, 186.

* TORDA M., J. MOLNÁR (1964): Boj proti trichofýciam hosp. zvierat. Slov. vydav. podohosp. lit., Bratislava.

TORRES G., L. K. GEORG (1956): A human case of Trichophyton gallinae infection. Arch. Derm. 74, 191.

VANBREUSEGHEM R. (1949): Description d'un nouveau dermatophyte isolé au Congo Belge, Sabouraudites (Microsporum) duboisii, n. sp. Ann. Parasit. 24, 252.

VANBREUSEGHEM R. (1949): La culture des dermatophytes in vitro sur des cheveux isolés. Ann. Parasit. 24, 559.

VANBREUSEGHEM R. (1950): Diagnose et systématique des dermatophytes. Contribution à la connaissance de teignes du Congo Belge. Ann. Soc. belge Méd. trop. 30, 865.

VANBREUSEGHEM R. (1963): Dermatophytes from the republic of Congo and Ruanda-Burundi, new description of Microsporum rivalieri. Sabouraudia 2, 215.

VARSAVSKY E., L. AJELLO (1964): The perfect and imperfect forms of a new keratino-philic fungus Arthroderma ciferrii sp. nov. Trichophyton georgii sp. nov. Riv. Pat. veget. III., 4, 351.

VRTIAK J., J. ZAPLETAL (1956): Trichophyton faviforme discoides — povodca oparu lysivého u hovädzieho dobytka. Vet. čas. 3, 204.

* VRTIAK J., Š. TKÁČIK, J. VODRÁŽKA (1962): Hubové ochorenia kože zvierat a boj proti nim. Slov. vydat. podohosp. lit., Bratislava.

WEITZMAN J. (1964): Variation in Microsporum gypseum. I. Genetic study of pleomor-phism. Sabouraudia 3, 195.

WERNER H. J., H. W. JOLLY, J. H. LEE (1964): Electron microscopic observations of Epidermophyton floccosum. J. invest. Derm. 43, 139.

WERNER H. J., H. W. JOLLY, B. O. SPURLOCK (1966): Electron microscope observations of the fine structure of Microsporum canis. J. invest. Derm. 46, 130.

* WILDFÜHR G. (1961): Medizinische Mikrobiologie, Immunologie und Epidemiologie. Teil II., VEB Georg Thieme, Leipzig.

ZIEGLER H., H. BÖHME (1963): Untersuchungen über den Haarabbau durch Dermatomy-zeten. Derm. Wschr. 148, 429.

GLOSSARY

abortive: incompletely developed

acrogenous: borne at the tip of a conidiophore

acropleurogenous: developing at the tip and along the sides

aleuries (aleuriospores): microconidia

anastomosis: hyphal fusion

anthropophilic: adapted for parasitic life and reproduction on man

apophysis: a swelling or a swollen filament

appendage: a filamentous process

arthrospore: a spore resulting from the breaking up of a hypha into cylindrical separate cells

ascigerous: having asci

ascigerous stage: perfect stage

ascocarp: a fruit body of the Ascomycetes

ascogenic:
ascogenous: ascus-producing

Ascomycetes: sac fungi

ascomycetous stage: perfect stage

ascospore: a spore borne in a sac-like cell called ascus

ascus: a spore sac in which nuclear fusion and meiosis precede spore formation in the *Ascomycetes*, usually containing 8 spores

asexual stage (state): — see imperfect stage

asteroid: with rays in star formation

basifugal: development in direction reverse to basipetal

basipetal: development in the direction towards the base, i.e. the apical part being oldest

catenulate: in chains

chandelier: candlestick-like or antler-like branched hyphae of dermatophytes

chlamydospore: thick-walled, asexual, intercalary, lateral or terminal cell containing stored food and capable of functioning as a spore

clavate: club-shaped

cleistothecium: a closed fruit body (*Ascomycetes*) without an ostiole, containing asci with ascospores

clubs: swollen hyphal tips

concurrent infection: simultaneous infection of other parts of the body caused by another dermatophyte

conidial stage: asexual, imperfect stage

conidiophore: more or less specialized hypha

conidium: spore borne externally in various ways

consecutive infection: designation for infection with other fungus species, secondarily isolated from a single lesion

coremia: bundles of hyphae (see synnema)

cottony: having a soft and cotton-like surface

decontamination: a method for excluding the growth of contaminating bacteria and nondermatophytic fungi

dermatophytes: a group of keratinophilous fungi capable of parasitizing homoiothermous animals

dermatophytosis: any disease caused by parasitic action of dermatophytes

dichotomous: bifurcation, forking

distal: remote from the point of origin

downy: having a fine, hairy appearance

ectothrix: forming spores outside the hair

eczema marginatum: special type of epidermophytia caused by *E. floccosum*

endoectothrix: dermatophytic elements both outside and inside the hair

endothrix: forming spores inside the hair

epidermophilic: adapted for parasitic life and reproduction in the epidermis

epidermophytia: special type of human dermatophytosis mostly caused by *E. floccosum*, *T. mentagrophytes* var. *interdigitale* and *T. rubrum*, involving intertriginous or unhaired areas

extrapillar: outside the hair

fascicle: a little group or bundle

favic: relating to a special type of dermatophytosis called favus or tinea favosa

faviform degeneration: a glabrous transformation of dermatophytic colony resembling a colony of favus incitant

favus: tinea favosa, a special type of dermatophytosis, in which scutula, yellowish crusts, develop around the hair base

ferrugineous: rusty

fertile: bearing spores

filament: a thread

floccose: cottony, in tufts

florentiform: producing abundant spores esp. conidia

fungemia: mycotic infection of the circulating blood, rare in dermatophytoses

fuseaux: macroconidia

fusiform: spindle-shaped

geophilic: adapted for saprophytic life and reproduction in the soil

germ tube: a germination hypha

glabrous: smooth

globose, globular: almost spherical

guttation: tear-like drops produced on the surface of the colony

hair-bait-method: Karling's method (isolation method based on the keratinophily) introduced by Vanbreuseghem into studies of dermatophytes

host: any animal or plant supporting a parasite

hypha: one of the threads of a mycelium

imperfect stage: asexual stage, a phase of the life cycle without sexual reproduction

inoculate: to introduce a microorganism or a substance containing microorganisms, into an organism or a substratum

in situ: in its natural position

intercalary: between two cells or hyphae

macroconidium: the larger conidium in those fungi which bear large and small spores

mentagre (French): tinea barbae

microconidium: the smaller conidium in those fungi which bear large and small spores

microfungi: fungi which do not produce large fruit bodies (yeasts and moulds)

microsporia: a special type of dermatophytosis caused by Microspora

mycelium: a mass of hyphae

mycemia: see fungemia

mycosis: a disease caused by parasitic fungi

nodular body: rounded mass of irregular shape composed of contorted and intertwined hyphae

ostiole: mouth, pore

pectinate: like the teeth of a comb

pedicel: small stalk

perfect stage: the portion of the life cycle in which spores are formed after nuclear fusion

peridium: the outer wall or limiting membrane of a fruit body

pleomorphic: cottony, sterile colony of dermatophyte, having two or more spore forms

pleurogenous: borne on the sides of a conidiophore

pseudocleistothecium: underdeveloped rudimentary cleistothecium without asci and ascospores

pyriform: pear-shaped

racquet hypha: a hypha with club-shaped cells, the clubbed end of one cell being attached to the small end of an adjacent cell

reproductive mycelium: mostly aerial mycelium producing spores

ringworm: tinea

rubriform: growing as a typical *T. rubrum*, i.e. a cottony, sterile colony

scutulum: a lenticular, yellowish crust formed at the base of the hair in tinea favosa

septate: having septa

septum: a cross wall

sessile: having no stem

sexual: having sex, resulting from fusion of gametes

spiral hypha: a hypha ending in a flat or helical coil

spore: a cell or cells differentiated for dissemination or reproduction (not only for survival as in bacteria!)

sporocarp: fruit body

sporophore: a spore producing and supporting structure

sterigma: a process from a cell supporting a spore

synnema: a group of hyphae sometimes joined together, generally upright and producing spores

thallospore: an asexual spore produced by septation of a hypha (e.g. an arthrospore)

tapering hyphae: peridial appendages

tinea: a term derived from the Latin word for worm. The round or serpentine-shaped lesions in the skin were thought to be caused by worms

tinea: ringworm

tinea barbae: beard ringworm

tinea capitis: scalp ringworm

tinea corporis: body ringworm

tinea cruris: groin ringworm

tinea favosa: favus, a special type of ringworm producing scutula, caused especially by *T. schoenleinii*, but also by *M. gypseum, T. violaceum, T. gallinae* (fowl favus), *T. mentagrophytes* var. *quinckeanum* (mouse favus)

tinea imbricata: a special type of ringworm in man caused by *T. concentricum*

tinea pedis: "athlete's foot", foot ringworm
tinea unguium: onychomycosis caused by dermatophytes
trichophytia: a special type of dermatophytosis caused by *Trichophyta*
verrucose: having small rounded processes or warts
zoophilic: adapted for parasitic life and reproduction on animals

INDEX TO THE NAMES OF SPECIES AND VARIETIES

The numerous printed in semibold-type refer to the first page of description of the principal species and varieties.

ERRATA

P. 7,   5th line:
         for 14 read 16

P. 8,   9th line:
         for infecting read contaminating

         14th line:
         for not attacking read which do not attack

P. 9,   10th line:
         for Infestation read Infection

         10th and 12th line:
         for 166 read 170

P. 10,   6th line:
         for man read animals

         8th line:
         for for the separation read division

         13th and 14th line:
         for macroconidial read macroconidia

P. 12,   4th line:
         read The distribution of dermatophytes on the Continents

         18th line:
         read The Auxiliary identification of dermatophytes by
         hair keratinolysis of various animals and man

         22nd line:
         for features read signs

P. 105, in the article *Microsporon cookei*:
         for Emm soil read Emmons

P. 212, left column, 3rd line from the end:
         for *Trichophyton kuehnii* read *Thallomicrosporon kuehnii*

         right column, 1st line from the end:
         for 614 read 164